Contact Lenses: Treatment Options for Ocular Disease

Contact Lenses
Treatment
Options for
Ocular Disease

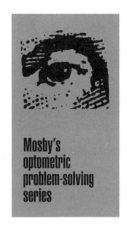

Mosby's
optometric
problem-solving
series

Edited by

Michael G. Harris
OD, JD, MS

Associate Dean
Clinical Professor
Chief, Contact Lens Clinic
School of Optometry
University of California, Berkeley
Berkeley, California

Series Editor

Richard London
MA, OD, FAAO

Diplomate in Binocular Vision and Perception
Pediatric and Rehabilitative Optometry
Oakland, California

with 12 contributors
with 68 illustrations

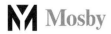 Mosby

St. Louis Baltimore Boston Carlsbad Chicago Naples New York Philadelphia Portland
London Madrid Mexico City Singapore Sydney Tokyo Toronto Wiesbaden

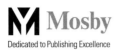

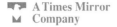

Dedicated to Publishing Excellence

A Times Mirror
Company

Executive Editor: Martha Sasser
Associate Developmental Editor: Amy Dubin
Project Manager: John Rogers
Production Editor: Jennifer Furey
Design Coordinator: Renée Duenow
Series Design: Jeanne Wolfgeher
Manufacturing Supervisor: Tony McAllister
Production: Carlisle Publishers Services

Printed in the United States of America
Composition by Carlisle Communications, Ltd.
Printing/binding by Maple-Vail Book Manufacturing Group

Mosby–Year Book, Inc.
11830 Westline Industrial Drive
St. Louis, Missouri 63146

International Standard Book Number 0-8151-4645-0

96 97 98 99 00 / 9 8 7 6 5 4 3 2 1

Contributors

Noel A. Brennan, MscOptom, PhD, FAAO, FVCO
Coles & Brennan Optometrists
Melbourne, Victoria
Australia

Nathan Efron, PhD, DSc
Professor of Clinical Optometry
Department of Optometry and Vision
Sciences
University of Manchester Institute of
Science and Technology
Manchester, United Kingdom

Cheslyn M. Gan, OD
Clinical Instructor
School of Optometry
University of California, Berkeley
Berkeley, California

Timothy J. Grant, BOptom, FAAO
Executive Director, Clinical and
Regulatory Affairs
Ciba Vision
Duluth, Georgia

Michael G. Harris, OD, JD, MS
Associate Dean
Clinical Professor
Chief, Contact Lens Clinic
School of Optometry
University of California, Berkeley
Berkeley, California

Brien A. Holden, PhD
Professor and Director
Cornea and Contact Lens Research Unit
School of Optometry
University of New South Wales
Kensington, New South Wales
Australia

Charles W. McMonnies, MS, FAAO
Visiting Professor
School of Optometry
University of New South Wales
Kensington, New South Wales
Australia

Kenneth A. Polse, OD, MS
Professor
School of Optometry
University of California, Berkeley
Berkeley, California

Reuben K. Rivera, OD

Research Optometrist
School of Optometry
University of California, Berkeley
Berkeley, California

Joel A. Silbert, OD, FAAO

Associate Professor of Optometry
Director, Cornea and Specialty Contact
Lens Service
The Eye Institute
Pennsylvania College of Optometry
Philadelphia, Pennsylvania

Robert Terry, BOptom

Principal Research Optometrist
Cornea and Contact Lens Research Unit
School of Optometry
University of New South Wales
Kensington, New South Wales
Australia

Frank Zisman, OD, PhD, FAAO

Associate Clinical Professor
Chief Vision Functions Clinic
Department of Optometry
University of California, Berkeley
Berkeley, California

To my family—
Dawn, Matt, Dan, Ashley, Lindsay,
to my parents,
and to the many contact lens practitioners
with whom I have worked over the years.

Preface

When contact lenses became popular in the 1950s, most practitioners and patients recognized only the cosmetic benefits of the marvelous devices. However, clinicians soon learned that contact lenses could be of great benefit in caring for patients with visual and ocular diseases. Unfortunately, they also found that when fitted without proper care, skill, and instructions, contact lenses could lead to ocular disease.

This book covers the integral relationship between contact lenses and ocular disease. Preventing adverse ocular effects when fitting contact lenses is a major challenge to all contact lens practitioners. Managing and treating ocular disease with specialized contact lenses is a difficult but extremely rewarding aspect of vision care.

The first five chapters of this text discuss visual or ocular disease processes and their relationship to contact lenses. Silbert discusses the causes and management of ocular infections in contact lens patients. McMonnies explains how tear deficiencies can affect contact lens wear. Grant, Terry, and Holden review the effects of soft extended-wear contact lenses on corneal physiology, while Polse, Rivera, and Gan discuss the complications associated with rigid gas-permeable extended lens wear. Zisman and Harris describe how therapeutically tinted contact lenses can help patients with various visual disorders.

In the final two chapters, Efron and Brennan describe specific visual and comfort problems associated with contact lens wear, that if untreated can lead to significant problems.

I hope the readers of this book will learn as much from the authors as I have. Each chapter contains valuable clinical insights into contact lens practice that knowledgeable and skillful practitioners will want to incorporate in their care of challenging contact lens patients.

Acknowledgments

I thank the authors and the staffs of their practices and institutions for their time and effort in writing the chapters for this text. My special thanks to Brenda Marshall, who assisted in the preparation of this book.

My thanks also to Series Editor Dr. Richard London, Kellie White, Amy Dubin, and the editorial production staff at Mosby for their assistance with this project.

Most importantly, I would like to thank my family, my friends, my colleagues, and my students for their love, friendship, and support.

Michael G. Harris
University of California, Berkeley

Contents

1

Microbial Infection in Contact Lens Wear

Joel A. Silbert

Key Terms

extended wear	blepharitis	*Acanthamoeba*
microbial infection	*Staphylococcus*	fungal keratitis
infectious keratitis	corneal ulcer	viral infection
noncompliance	*Pseudomonas*	

Are contact lenses prescription medical devices to be regularly monitored on the eye, or are they simply trivialized, boxed products to be bought off the shelf of a supermarket pharmacy or from a toll-free mail-order number? Although this debate is still raging, it should be clear that advances in contact lens material and design have not eliminated the risk of infection or other complications of lens wear. Frank infection from contact lens wear is not common, but complications can and do occur with lens wear. In addition to problems associated with lens care systems and spoilage, physiological problems such as corneal edema, staining, and hyperemia are frequently found. Pathological changes including corneal vascularization, infiltration, and abrasion are less commonly seen but do occur, but the practitioner generally manages these satisfactorily with minimal permanent tissue damage. Corneal infection, although rare, carries with it such severe consequences as major tissue damage and permanent vision loss that the practitioner must vigilantly observe for these signs in both symptomatic and asymptomatic patients. Patients and providers need to keep uppermost in their minds not just the visual and cosmetic enhancements attendant with contact lens wear, but also the responsibilities and risks associated with their use.

Even when eye care professionals exercise the greatest care, contact lens patients may develop complications from their own noncompliance with recommended procedures and lens care products. Other complications may arise from inherent problems with the immune system's functionality, dermatological conditions adversely affecting the patient's lids, lashes, and meibomian glands, or the tear film's status. Complications may ensue secondary to lens use under less than favorable conditions such as with extended wear, or in contaminated environments, or from use of topical medications or harsh preservatives. Indeed, the contact lens should be viewed as an ocular health care device capable of providing not only great improvement in visual efficiency but also great harm if treated cavalierly.

Fortunately, few disorders among the many known complications associated with contact lens wear are actually sight threatening. Much of the eye care provider's time is spent managing and educating patients about complications that although vexing to both practitioner and patient are rarely associated with vision loss (for example, dry eye symptoms, solution-related sensitivity, or contact–lens-related papillary conjunctivitis). Much less frequently encountered, the patient who develops an eye infection from either lens-related or non–lens-related causes may experience complications ranging from chronic problems to acute ocular challenges so virulent that vision may permanently be lost within a matter of days.

Contact Lens Complications

Sight Threatening
Ulcerative bacterial keratitis
Fungal keratitis
Acanthamoeba keratitis
Contact lens superior limbic keratoconjunctivitis
Corneal vascularization
Severe corneal distortion

Not Sight Threatening
Corneal edema (hypoxia)
Giant papillary conjunctivitis
Corneal abrasion/3–9 o'clock staining
Superficial punctate keratitis
Solution toxicity/hypersensitivity

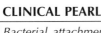

Contact Lens Complications—cont'd

Inflammation/infiltrates
Hyperemia/tight lens reaction
Epithelial microcysts
Endothelial polymegethism
Dellen formation
Dimple veiling
Pseudodendrites
Refractive changes/corneal "molding"

Factors Influencing Microbial Infection

As previously noted, contact–lens-related infectious keratitis is rare. Large-scale studies of cosmetic hydrogel extended wear have shown an annualized incidence rate of approximately 0.2%.[1,2] In addition, case-control studies have repeatedly pointed out the increased risk of corneal infection with hydrogel extended wear, compared with rigid and hydrogel daily wear. The risk of infectious keratitis among users of cosmetic hydrogel extended-wear lenses is estimated to be between 2 and 15 times that seen with daily-wear hydrogel lens use.[3-6]

The hydrogel lens' widespread use presents a formidable challenge to the prevention of infection for a variety of reasons. First, the gel lens provides an excellent substrate for biofilms that adhere rapidly to its surfaces. Bacterial attachment to biofilm is a well-established phenomenon not unique to contact lenses.[7,8] This reservoir of bacteria adhering to lens surfaces provides a pool of potential pathogens that can breach the cornea's defense barriers in the presence of epithelial compromise.[7]

CLINICAL PEARL

Bacterial attachment to biofilm provides a reservoir of potential pathogens that may breach corneal defenses in the presence of epithelial compromise.

Although corneal infection may occur in daily-wear and extended-wear patients, the preponderance of ulcers affects the extended-wear hydrogel candidate.[9] Repeated anoxic stress to the cornea with extended wear causes changes in every layer of the cornea, including epithelial staining and microcysts, increased epithelial fragility and reduced epithelial adhesion, stromal edema and thinning, and endothelial polymegethism.[10,11] Other factors in addition to chronic hypoxia exist that may foster contact–lens-related infection. These include manipulative trauma to the corneal epithelium[12]; disruption of eyelid wiping/cleansing action in hydrogel extended wear[13]; use of contaminated solutions, cases, and cosmetics[11]; and concurrent topical steroid use.[14] Topical steroids predispose to corneal microbial infection by suppressing immune defense mechanisms, facilitating infection, and masking its severity. Additional factors include blepharitis and diabetes. Diabetes mellitus is a risk factor for infectious keratitis, particularly in extended wear.[15,16] The diabetic eye has systemic abnormalities (including poorer healing), and exhibits greater corneal epithelial fragility.[17]

The low incidence of ocular infection with contact lenses points to the highly effective defense mechanisms of the cornea and outer eye. In particular, the antimicrobial functions afforded by normal tear constituents, such as lysozyme, lactoferrins, immunoglobulins, and beta-lysin, control the microbial load in the tear film, especially that introduced by lens handling in daily-wear users.[18]

Disposable extended-wear lenses, often recommended for the reduction of problems caused by noncompliance, papillary conjunctivitis, and age-related changes in lenses, have been associated with ulcerative bacterial keratitis.[5,6] Although disposable lenses may reduce some lens-related complications, hypoxia is believed to be the primary factor in the development of ulcerative keratitis in wearers of disposable extended-wear soft lenses.[19-21]

Noncompliance with lens care is integral to the development of contact–lens-related infections. Anecdotal reports abound of patients incorrectly storing lenses in saline rather than in disinfecting solutions. How many patients are truly compliant with proper lens care techniques as described in Mondino et al's definition of compliance?[9]

1. Hand washing before handling lenses
2. Use of FDA-approved care system according to manufacturer's guidelines and with appropriate hygiene
3. Close following of prescribed lens-wearing schedule
4. Absence of microbial contamination of lens solutions and cases

Contamination of lens care solutions may be an important source of infecting microbes in contact–lens-related ulcerative keratitis. Nevertheless, case-controlled studies have not identified noncompliance with normal lens care as a requisite risk factor[6] and such a mechanism needs further study. Indeed, if this route were a primary one, we should expect a much higher incidence of infection among users of daily-wear lenses because contact between contaminated solutions and lenses occurs with much greater frequency in this mode of wear.[13]

Nevertheless, all offices involved in fitting and dispensing contact lenses should provide appropriate ongoing education for patients and office staff regarding lens care and hygiene. This means not only adherence to recommended lens cleaning and disinfection procedures, but also recognition of the need for hand washing before manipulation of the eye or contact lens. Practitioners need to query their patients on each visit about their lens care techniques and the specific products used in lens care. It is remarkable how often patients lapse in appropriate lens hygiene, most often in their shocking use of saline instead of prescribed disinfecting solutions and in their lack of lens rubbing with surfactant cleaners before disinfection and storage. This, unfortunately, has been observed more frequently since the advent of disposable lenses, indicating patients' faulty association of disposable contact lenses with freedom from risks of complications.[22] Patient education and reeducation need to be incorporated in the office protocol. Educating patients to remove their extended-wear lenses at prescribed intervals, to clean and disinfect lenses at appropriate intervals, and to clean and air-dry contact lens cases will reduce risks of contact lens infection.[23]

The Symptomatic Patient

The clinician must always maintain a high degree of suspicion when examining a contact lens patient presenting with a red, irritated, or painful eye. Complaints of ocular irritation (especially when expressed by a contact lens patient calling the office) must not be ignored, and the patient should be seen promptly. A patient with an irritated or painful eye, whether intensely hyperemic or white and quiet, deserves an immediate and thorough evaluation. Complaints of photophobia, particularly in an eye that was previously quiescent, should be viewed with alarm because this sign of inflammation may be a harbinger of corneal infection.

The clinician will want to evaluate the symptomatic patient to rule out blepharitis or conjunctivitis and institute therapy as indicated. The practitioner should include lid eversion to rule out embedded foreign bodies, a displaced or folded lens, or contact–lens-induced papillary conjunctivitis. Disclosing agents such as sodium fluorescein and rose bengal are useful to identify the presence of corneal abrasions, "lost" hydrogel lenses, epithelial erosions or defects, and manifestations of dry eye.

An acutely inflamed or painful eye in a previously asymptomatic contact lens wearer must be viewed as a potential corneal infection and an ophthalmic urgency. If a nonulcerative keratitis is diagnosed, as, for example, from solution toxicity (BAK or hydrogen peroxide) or a viral keratitis, lens wear should be discontinued and the patient managed supportively until resolution allows resumption of lens wear. With corneal ulcers of presumed infectious origin, however, the clinician should look for hallmark signs of epithelial defect with underlying stromal infiltration. Anterior chamber reaction and purulent discharge may be present. The clinician should obtain corneal scrapings for cultures and stains before initiating antibiotic therapy.[24] The patient's contact lenses, carrying cases, and solutions can be cultured to help identify the causative agent. Aggressive broad-spectrum antibiotic therapy should be initiated immediately after cultures have been taken, with clinical suspicion focused on the worst case scenario of *P. aeruginosa* infection until proven otherwise.[25] Based on the clinical presentation the practitioner will determine whether the patient can be effectively managed in the office setting, should be referred to a corneal specialist for continued management, or should be hospitalized. The latter course is often followed with severe or unresponsive ulcerative keratitis and with noncompliant patients.[26]

Staphylococcal Blepharitis

Contact lens candidates should be examined for evidence of staphylococcal blepharitis, because this chronic lid disorder can lead to significant corneal complications, including ulcerative keratitis.[23] The patient with blepharitis has a higher than normal bacterial load on the lid margins, in the tear film, and on the ocular surface. With contact lens wear influencing the physiological environment, patients with blepharitis are poorly tolerant of contact lenses. Although most cases of blepharitis among the contact–lens-wearing population are caused by staphylococci, blepharitis also may be caused by seborrhea, dry eye, acne rosacea, *Demodex folliculorum,* and *Phthiriasis palpebrum* (pubic lice infestation of the cilia).[27] Both *S. aureus* and *S. epidermidis* (common gram-positive bacteria resident in the skin and eyelids) have been associated with corneal infection in contact lens wearers and nonwearers. *S. epidermidis* is part of the skin's normal flora, but may infect the cornea through self-transmittal, as, for example, when patients handle lenses and lens cases.[23] It is frequently implicated in ulcerative keratitis in prolonged wear of bandage hydrogel lenses[28] and in infections associated with contaminated eye cosmetics.[29] *S. aureus* also is self-transmitted, is a cause of both blepharitis and conjunctivitis, and is highly associated with marginal corneal infiltrates as part of a hypersensitivity reaction. In blepharitis caused by either organism the lid margins are typically inflamed and hyperemic. A crusty yellow exudate often encloses the base of the lashes (Figure 1-1). Long-term lid disease may lead to thickened and irregular lid margins, and areas of misdirected lashes or lash loss. Patients with chronic staphylococcal blepharitis also are prone to recurrent hordeola and chalazia. The staphylococci are almost always the etiological agents, leading to a focal infection of either the meibomian gland within the tarsal plate area (internal hordeolum or meibomitis) or the glands of Zeis or Moll near the eyelid margin (external hordeolum) (Figure 1-2).

When a stye or hordeolum is present, frequent applications of moist hot compresses supplemented with an antibiotic ointment (bacitracin, polysporin, or erythromycin) rubbed into the lid margin

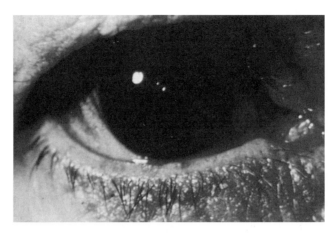

FIGURE 1-1 Chronic staphylococcal blepharitis with crusty exudate enclosing the base of the lashes.

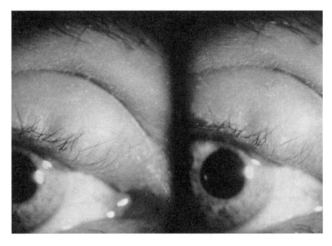

FIGURE 1-2 Internal hordeolum leading to meibomitis. If poorly drained, it will ultimately become a granulomatous chalazion.

are usually effective. Antibiotic therapy should be continued for several days following the acute stage. A chalazion may develop as a local immune granulomatous response to a poorly drained hordeolum. The patient typically complains about a small nodular lump in the lid that may be quiescent or inflamed. Chalazia are best managed with prompt and frequent applications of moist hot compresses and topical antibiotic-steroid combination ointment. Large and nonresponsive chalazia are best treated with triamcinolone injections (directly into the granuloma) or with excision and drainage.

Symptoms of staphylococcal lid disease vary widely and include foreign body sensation and burning, worse upon waking. Patients with chronic staphylococcal blepharitis also are prone to the hypersensitivity effects of bacterial exotoxins that build up in the inferior cul-de-sac during sleep. A local inflammatory response to these toxins can cause inferior punctate corneal stippling, sterile marginal corneal infiltration, micropannus, phlyctenulosis, and a weepy eczema at the lateral lid fornices with associated skin excoriation and angular conjunctivitis[30] (Figures 1-3 and 1-4). Topical steroids (typically prescribed as steroid-antibiotic combinations) are helpful when signs of staphylococcal toxin hypersensitivity are present.

If chronic staphylococcal blepharitis is diagnosed, the clinician should be conservative in prescribing contact lenses with infected patients because lens wear may exacerbate the underlying condition and facilitate vascularization and corneal infection. In general, these patients should use an optical correction other than contact lenses. Patients demonstrating minimal lid disease without hypersensitivity and who are willing to employ regular lid hygiene (lid scrubs) may achieve some success using rigid gas-permeable (RGP) contact lenses.

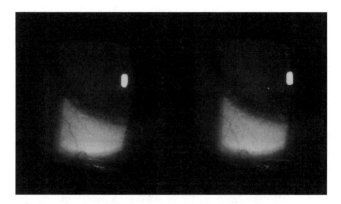

FIGURE 1-3 Inferior corneal staining caused by staphylococcal exotoxins.

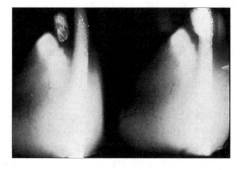

FIGURE 1-4 Inferior corneal micropannus, a hypersensitivity response to staphylococcal exotoxin.

RGP lenses are more easily cleaned and are less prone to the effects of bacterial adherence than hydrogels. Extended wear of any lens (hydrogel or rigid) should be strictly avoided.

Ulcerative Bacterial Keratitis

Ulcerative keratitis is the most severe complication associated with contact lens wear. Although not commonly seen in normal healthy eyes, the incidence of ulcerative keratitis has markedly increased with the growing popularity of contact lenses over the past two decades (in particular with extended wear of hydrogel lenses). As many as 66% of cases of ulcerative keratitis seen in major eye referral centers in the United States and United Kingdom are contact lens related.[4] As we have seen, the use of extended-wear hydrogel lenses is a significant risk factor for corneal ulcers compared to rigid or daily-wear hydrogel lenses. This risk increases with consecutive nights of extended wear.[3,6]

An infectious corneal ulcer is an epithelial defect involving tissue erosion and necrosis into the stroma with associated corneal infiltration (Figure 1-5). Infiltrates are aggregates of whitish inflammatory cells that have migrated to the infection site via the tears or through the cornea from limbal vessels in response to chemotactic stimuli from the damaged corneal tissue. The majority of inflammatory cells making up corneal infiltrates are polymorphonuclear leukocytes, but macrophages and lymphocytes also are included.

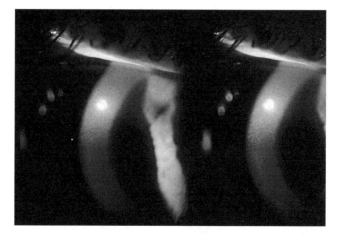

FIGURE 1-5 Ulcerative keratitis caused by *S. aureus*. Note the focally concentrated and well-demarcated infiltrates with surrounding corona of white blood cells. Staining with sodium fluorescein reveals an overlying epithelial defect.

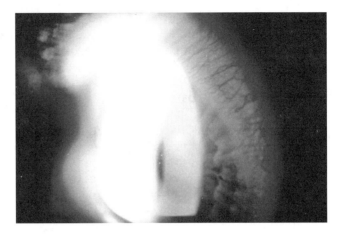

FIGURE 1-6 Staphylococcal ulcerative keratitis. Note the grayish-white concentrated infiltration with overlying epithelial defect. The rest of the cornea remains clear.

The most commonly cultured organisms in contact–lens-related ulcerative keratitis, in descending frequency, follow[31,32]:

1. *Pseudomonas aeruginosa*
2. *Staphylococcus aureus*
3. *Staphylococcus epidermidis*
4. *Streptococcus pneumoniae*
5. Beta-hemolytic streptococcus
6. *Serratia marcescens*

Infectious staphylococcal ulcers typically present as zones of well-demarcated white or pale yellow infiltrates with an overlying epithelial defect (Figure 1-6). *S. aureus* may produce infectious ulcers that are centrally or paracentrally located, or may produce marginal, allergic, sterile ulcers that are caused by hypersensitivity reactions to released exotoxins.

Pseudomonas aeruginosa has been identified as the major pathogen in as many as two thirds of cases of hydrogel extended-wear infectious keratitis,[33,34] and is capable of producing devastating corneal complications. This gram-negative rod lives in moist environments and is commonly found in sinks, cosmetics, eye drop bottles, and distilled water containers used by patients preparing their own saline. It cannot penetrate the intact corneal epithelium, but can quickly necrotize corneal tissue after a break in the epithelial surface has occurred. Because *Pseudomonas* can and does adhere to soft lens surfaces, alterations to the corneal epithelium induced by hypoxia and other risk factors can facilitate invasion and infection, most notably in extended wear of hydrogel lenses. Its greatest danger stems from its release of proteoglycanase, endotoxins, and exotoxins that can cause rapid corneal melting even after bacterial death from antibiosis.[35]

CLINICAL PEARL

The greatest danger from Pseudomonas *corneal infection stems from its release of proteoglycanase, endotoxins, and exotoxins that can cause rapid corneal necrosis even after bacterial death from antibiosis.*

A *Pseudomonas* ulcer is usually centrally located with a large epithelial defect overlying a dense stromal infiltrate. Hypopyon is often seen in the anterior chamber floor (Figure 1-7). The cornea becomes edematous, and mucoidal, purulent material often clings to the ulcer.

The clinician should always consider ulcerative keratitis associated with contact lens wear to be potentially caused by *Pseudomonas*. The risk of this organism being found in positive cultures is high in the hydrogel-wearing population and insufficient treatment can have catastrophic results. The size and location of corneal ulcers are highly variable and are not good indicators of pathogenicity, especially because all corneal infections start out as small lesions. Thus it is best to assume that any corneal ulcer might be the most pathogenic. After corneal scrapings are completed, initial therapy should be broad spectrum with excellent coverage of gram-negative organisms. The therapeutic goal is to eradicate pathogenic microbes quickly, reduce the damage caused by inflammation, and foster corneal reepithelialization. Traditional antibiotic therapies for presumed ulcerative bacterial keratitis use commercial strength and fortified cephalosporins and aminoglycosides. Fortified topical antibiotics provide greater drug concentration, contact time, and penetration; they are prepared by combining parenteral antibiotic with artificial tears to achieve the desired concentration.[36] More recently, the use of topical fluoroquinolones to treat ulcerative bacterial keratitis in compliant patients has been gaining favor among clinicians.

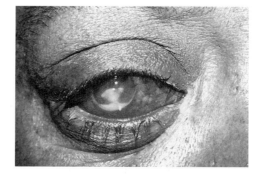

FIGURE 1-7 *Pseudomonas aeruginosa* corneal ulcer in a patient using extended-wear hydrogel lenses. Note large central corneal defect and stromal infiltration with hypopyon and inherent discharge.

Patients often wish to return to lens wear as soon as their eyes are no longer red and irritation is absent. The clinician must closely monitor the patient during the healing phase, maintaining antibiosis and adjunct therapies until all signs of infection are gone, with complete reepithelialization of the ulcer.[37] A suitable period of time should elapse in which no lenses are worn even after signs of infection resolve. A return to extended wear should be discouraged. Fresh lenses should be used with a new lens case and fresh solutions. The patient should discard opened solutions and used lens cases. A complete review of lens care should be undertaken, and close monitoring of the patient's wearing schedule and physiological response as lens wear resumes is essential.[37]

Acanthamoeba Keratitis

A relatively rare but catastrophic corneal infection seen with greater frequency among contact lens wearers in recent years is caused by Acanthamoeba. The first reported cases involving contact lens wear occurred in 1985 among healthy soft lens wearers using homemade saline solutions.[38] Since that time several hundred cases have been reported, with the majority of cases occurring among contact lens wearers who prepare saline from distilled water and salt tablets, and among individuals exposed to contaminated water sources while wearing soft lenses.[39,40]

Acanthamoebae are free-living protozoans found in soil, air, sewage, tap and well water, swimming pools and hot tubs, lakes, and sea water.[31] Most Acanthamoeba infections have been found among patients using daily-wear hydrogel lenses, but there have been reports of Acanthamoeba keratitis in users of extended-wear soft lenses, rigid gas- permeable lenses, and Saturn lenses.[38,41,42] The organisms have been observed adhering to the contact lenses of keratitis patients and have been recovered from lens cases of symptomatic and asymptomatic patients; it therefore appears that the organism's adherence to the lens is a likely vehicle by which it is inoculated onto the corneal surface.[43]

Acanthamoeba normally lives as a vegetative mobile trophozoite. However, if the amoeba is challenged by its environment or pharmacologically, it changes into a double-walled cyst, which accounts for its resistance to drug therapy. The organism can survive in chlorinated pools, hot tubs, and even in dry environments, all of which are potential modes of transmission.[44]

Studies have shown that thermal disinfection is highly effective against the trophozoite and cyst forms of pathogenic species of Acanthamoeba.[45,46] Chemical disinfection systems, on the other hand (including hydrogen peroxide), have shown variable efficacy in killing pathogenic strains of Acanthamoeba when used in commercially available forms.[47-49] Perhaps the best response is to recognize that contact lens disinfection systems depend on the "contribution of elements." As such, digitally rubbing lenses is important in reducing the volume of organisms on lens surfaces. The use of a cysticidal, alcohol-based surfactant cleaner and an FDA-approved chemical disinfection system should be effective for hydrogel lens users.[49]

Patients should be discouraged from swimming in any type of water while wearing contact lenses or from rinsing their lenses in tap or other nonsterile water sources before lens placement. Clinicians should recommend thermal disinfection for patients at risk for such exposure. Practitioners and staff should take the precaution of cleaning trial lenses and their patients' lenses that were removed for in-office modifications with an alcohol-based cleaner before reinserting them.

Early infection with *Acanthamoeba* in a contact lens wearer may lead to signs and symptoms of varying intensities. A lens wearer presenting with conjunctival hyperemia, tearing, punctate staining, and some discomfort is not a rare phenomenon. In the absence of epithelial trauma many cases are mistaken in these early stages for herpes simplex keratitis because nonspecific punctate keratopathy and pseudodendritic lesions often are present.[50] A dendritiform pattern that may be mistaken for a h. simplex dendrite is seen in "elevated epithelial lines," which have been shown to contain actively migrating trophozoites.[51] If epithelial trauma has occurred in lens wearers exposed to contaminated fluids, inflammatory and infectious signs rapidly become evident. These signs include folliculosis, stromal and ring infiltration, hypopyon, uveitis, scleritis, and corneal melt[52] (Figures 1-8 and 1-9).

A patient with *Acanthamoeba* keratitis may experience ocular pain totally out of proportion to the clinical picture.[53] This may be caused by stromal keratoneuritis or by scleritis with optic disc edema.[39]

A correct diagnosis of *Acanthamoeba* infection often is made after attempts to treat initially suspected bacterial or viral infections have failed. Corneal scrapings and cultures are essential whenever evidence

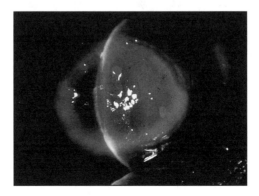

FIGURE 1-8 *Acanthamoeba* keratitis with severe corneal melt and endotoxin-induced ring infiltrate.

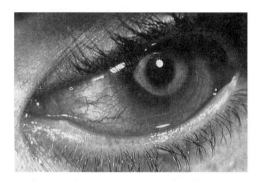

FIGURE 1-9 Late-stage *Acanthamoeba* keratitis with pronounced ring infiltrate. Severe vision loss will require penetrating keratoplasty in most cases.

indicates microbial keratitis. However, these may be negative if *Acanthamoeba* has migrated to the stroma. Furthermore, the protozoa might be present but overlooked in a culture positive for *Pseudomonas*.[54] Laboratory tests to help identify *Acanthamoeba* infection include staining techniques, cell cultures, impression cytology, and direct and indirect fluorescein antibody testing.[52] If scrapings fail to produce organisms, corneal biopsy may become necessary, although current specular microscopy techniques can identify the organisms in the stroma and avoid biopsy.

A variety of antifungal agents administered topically and systemically are used in medical therapy[55] in addition to antibiotics and corticosteroids. Cases recognized early frequently respond to treatment with polyhexamethylene biguanide 0.02%. However, medical cures are often unsuccessful because *Acanthamoeba* is highly resistant to pharmacological agents and because of delays in treatment resulting from late recognition of the cause. Many cases require penetrating keratoplasty and some of these will require repeat grafts because the infection may recur in the grafted tissue.

Given the poor outcome of medical therapy and the devastating visual consequences attendant with *Acanthamoeba* infection, the contact lens practitioner's best weapons against this pathogen are education and prevention. Constant reinforcement of proper lens care and hygiene with particular emphasis on avoiding lens immersion in nonsterile water is essential.

CLINICAL PEARL

Given the poor outcome of medical therapy and the devastating visual consequences that are attendant with Acanthamoeba *infection, the contact lens practitioner's best weapons against this pathogen are education and prevention.*

Fungal Keratitis

Fungal keratitis (keratomycosis) is a rare complication of contact lens wear that has been seen with greater frequency over the past 20 years with the increasing use of topical corticosteroids.[56] A recent retrospective study conducted at the Bascom Palmer Eye Institute in southern Florida reported on 125 cases of fungal keratitis from 1982 to 1992.[57] The risk factors for fungal keratitis in this study were as shown in the box below.

Risk Factors for Fungal Keratitis

Trauma (44.0%)
Chronic topical pharmaceutical agents (12.8%)
Diabetes mellitus (12.0%)
Topical corticosteroids (7.2%)
Extended wear/bandage lenses (5.6%)
Metallic foreign body (4.0%)
Penetrating keratoplasty (3.2%)
Systemic disease (non-diabetes) (3.2%)
Anterior uveitis (2.4%)
H. simplex keratitis (1.6%)
H. zoster keratitis (1.6%)
Radial keratotomy (0.8%)
Vernal conjunctivitis (0.8%)
Systemic corticosteroids (0.8%)

(Modified from Rosa RH, Miller D, Alfonso EC. The changing spectrum of fungal keratitis in south Florida, *Ophthalmol* 101:1005–1013, 1994).

The fungi are nonmotile plantlike organisms growing as single-cell yeasts or multicellular molds; yeasts are the most common fungi cultured from normal conjunctivae.[58] Most of the fungi that cause keratomycosis produce opportunistic corneal infections in immuno-suppressed or immunocompromised eyes.[59] The yeast responsible for most fungal infections is *Candida albicans*[60]; *Fusarium* is the most common filamentous genus.[61] *Aspergillus* also is a common pathogen involved in fungal infections.[60]

Even among contact lens wearers, fungi are not considered part of the normal ocular flora,[58] but can contaminate lens cases, solutions, and "spare" (old) lenses (Figures 1-10 and 1-11).

Fungal spoilation rates of worn extended-wear lenses have been reported from 2% to 41%.[56,62] In a large series of culture-proven fungal ulcerative keratitis cases, Wilhelmus et al[56] found that *Fusarium* and other filamentous fungi were responsible for infections involving

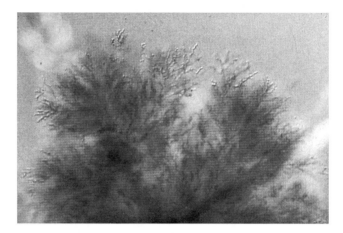

FIGURE 1-10 Branching filamentous hyphae of a fungally contaminated soft contact lens. (Courtesy Dr. R Weisbarth.)

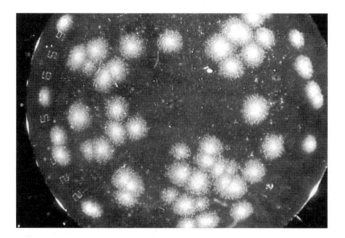

FIGURE 1-11 Yeast colonies growing on a contaminated soft contact lens. (Courtesy Dr. R Weisbarth.)

cosmetic hydrogel lenses, whereas yeasts such as *Candida* were responsible for infections involving therapeutic or bandage hydrogel lenses.

Many fungi can adhere to and invade the matrix of hydrogel lens polymers, particularly when lenses are worn and deposited.[63,64] Thermal disinfection has proven the most reliable means of preventing fungal spoilage of soft contact lenses, although spores can survive the heating cycle.[56] Many cold storage disinfection systems are weak in their ability to kill fungal pathogens and often require long soaking periods to do so. A minimum of a 45-minute to 60-minute soak in 3% hydrogen peroxide has been recommended to render fungal pathogens inactive.[65]

Fungal corneal ulcers vary in their presentation and course depending on the organism and the host's immunological status. Ulcers can be chronic and slowly progressive or acute and virulent. Clinical appearance may include conjunctival injection, epithelial defects, gray corneal surface, anterior uveitis, feathery defect borders, raised infiltrates, and satellite lesions.[57]

Antifungal agents commonly used to treat fungal ulcers include natamycin, amphotericin B, miconazole, ketaconazole, and clotrimazole. Adjunct therapy includes topical cycloplegia and agents to lower intraocular pressure (if elevated from inflammation).[59] Treatment of fungal ulcers is difficult and topical therapies may be ineffective, thus requiring surgical debridement, conjunctival flaps, and even penetrating keratoplasty.[59]

Fungal ulcers are uncommon in contact–lens-wearing patients and can be avoided through attention to the suggestions listed in the box below.

How to Avoid Fungal Ulcers

1. Wash hands before handling lenses.
2. Avoid using distilled water for lens rinsing or preparation of enzyme solutions.
3. Do not use homemade saline solution.
4. Use approved lens cleaners and disinfectants on a daily basis; rub lenses with cleaners before placing in disinfectant solutions.
5. If using hydrogen peroxide disinfectants, use longer exposure time (45 to 60 minutes) before neutralization.
6. Replace lens cases frequently.
7. Do not keep old lenses; store spare lenses in approved chemical disinfectant and replace solutions at least once a month.
8. Discard any lens that has a suspicious appearance.

Viral Infections

Although they are not true complications of contact lens wear, viral infections are common in the general population and will affect contact lens wearers with about the same frequency. Both adenoviral and herpetic corneal infections will occasionally be observed by contact lens practitioners. The adenoviral infections cause great discomfort for patients, especially in epidemic keratoconjunctivitis (EKC), in which the cornea may develop diffuse epithelial staining followed by long-lasting subepithelial infiltrates. The presence of folliculosis and lymphadenopathy is often helpful in differentiating between viral and non-viral etiologies in contact lens wearers (Figure 1-12). The herpes

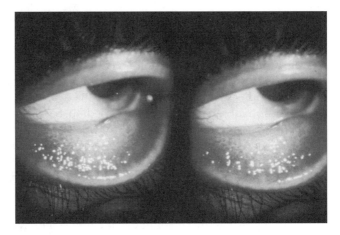

FIGURE 1-12 Pronounced folliculosis seen with EKC and other viral infections. Giant follicles on the upper palpebral conjunctiva that may be caused by *Chlamydia* must be differentiated from contact–lens-induced papillae.

simplex virus is not uncommon and recurrent infections often lead to the development of a true dendrite. Herpes simplex, however, is a great mimicker, and classic herpetic dendritic corneal lesions may not be immediately evident. Other conditions can create a dendritiform lesion that may resemble a herpetic dendrite when the lesion is actually a pseudodendrite (e.g., raised epithelial lines in *Acanthamoeba* infection).[66]

HIV (or human immunodeficiency virus) has been isolated from the blood, semen, vaginal secretions, and tears of infected patients.[67] No documented reports have implicated tears as a vector of transmission or indicated that the disease can be spread by contact with contact lenses or ocular secretions other than blood. This is probably because of the extremely low levels of HIV that exist in tears and the conjunctival epithelium.[68] HIV is a fragile virus and cannot survive long out of the body. Experimental evidence has shown that when HIV is inoculated into contact lenses both heat and cold disinfection systems are effective in killing it.[69] Nevertheless, all eye care personnel should use universal precautions and disposable gloves when examining HIV-positive patients or if there are cuts, scratches, or lesions on the examiner's hands. All office instruments and diagnostic contact lenses must be disinfected between patients according to published Centers for Disease Control and Prevention (CDC) guidelines. For disinfection of soft lenses, the CDC recommends thermal disinfection (172° F to 176° F for 10 minutes) or use of a commercially available hydrogen peroxide disinfection system. Rigid contact lenses are to be disinfected in 3% hydrogen peroxide using the same protocols as with soft lenses.[70]

Conclusion

When examining a contact lens patient, the practitioner must always maintain a high degree of clinical suspicion for signs and symptoms of infection. At every opportunity it is important to reinforce patient education, monitor compliance with approved lens care systems, and influence patient decisions regarding modes of lens wear to reduce conditions that make the patient more susceptible to infection. When evidence of infection is found, however, the clinician must assume an aggressive posture in making arrangements for prompt and appropriate referral or in instituting therapy and management, if the potentially devastating effects of microbial infection are to be minimized.

> **CLINICAL PEARL**
>
> *At every opportunity it is important to reinforce patient education, monitor compliance, and influence patient decisions regarding modes of lens wear to reduce conditions that make the patient more susceptible to infection.*

References

1. Poggio EC, Glynn RJ, Schein OD, et al: The incidence of ulcerative keratitis among users of extended-wear soft contact lenses, *N Engl J Med* 321:779, 1989.
2. MacRae S, Herman C, Stulting D, et al: Corneal ulcer and adverse reaction rates in premarket contact lens studies, *Am J Ophthalmol* 111:457, 1991.
3. Schein OD, Glynn RJ, Poggio EC, et al: The relative risk of ulcerative keratitis among users of daily-wear and extended-wear soft contact lenses, *N Engl J Med* 321:773, 1989.
4. Dart JG, Stapleton F, Minassian D: Contact lenses and other risk factors in microbial keratitis, *Lancet* 338:651, 1991.
5. Buehler PO, Schein OD, Stamler JF, et al: The increased risk of ulcerative keratitis among disposable soft contact lens users, *Arch Ophthalmol* 110:1555, 1992.
6. Matthews TD, Frazer DG, Minassian DC, et al: Risks of keratitis and patterns of use with disposable contact lenses, *Arch Ophthalmol* 110:1559, 1992.
7. Stern GA, Zam ZS: The pathogenesis of contact lens-associated *Pseudomonas aeruginosa* corneal ulceration: I. The effect of contact lens coatings on adherence of *Pseudomonas aeruginosa* to soft contact lenses, *Cornea* 5:41-45, 1987.
8. Slusher MM, Myrvik QN, Lewis JC, et al: Extended wear lenses, biofilm, and bacterial adhesion, *Arch Ophthalmol* 105:110-115, 1987.
9. Mondino BJ, Weissman BA, Farb MD, et al: Corneal ulcers associated with daily-wear and extended-wear contact lenses, *Am J Ophthalmol* 102:58-65, 1986.
10. Holden BA, Sweeney DF, Vannas A, et al: Effects of long-term extended contact lens wear on the human cornea, *Inv Ophthalmol Vis Sci* 26:1489-1501, 1985.
11. Chalupa EC, Swarbrick HA, Holden BA, et al: Severe corneal infections associated with contact lens wear, *Ophthalmol* 94(1):17-22, 1987.
12. Galentine PG, Cohen EJ, Laibson PR, et al: Corneal ulcers associated with extended-wear lenses, *Arch Ophthalmol* 102:891, 1984.
13. Swarbrick HA, Holden BA: Complications of Hydrogel Extended Wear Lenses. In Silbert JA (ed): *Anterior Segment Complications of Contact Lens Wear*, New York, 1994, Churchill Livingstone, 289-316.

14. Stern GA, Lubniewski A, Allen C: The interaction between *Pseudomonas aeruginosa* and the corneal epithelium, *Arch Ophthalmol* 103:1221, 1985.

15. Eichenbaum JW, Feldstein M, Podos SM: Extended wear aphakic soft contact lenses and corneal ulcers, *Br J Ophthalmol* 66:663, 1982.

16. Spoor TC, Hartel WC, Wynn P, Spoor DK: Complications of continuous wear soft contact lenses in a non-referral population, *Arch Ophthalmol* 102:1312, 1984.

17. Millidot M, O'Leary DJ: Abnormal epithelial fragility in diabetes and contact lens wear, *Acta Ophthalmol* 59:827, 1981.

18. Mowrey-McKee MF, Sampson HJ, Proskin HM: Microbial contamination of hydrophilic contact lenses. Part II: Quantification of microbes after patient handling and after aseptic removal from the eye, *CLAO* 18:240, 1992.

19. Killingsworth DW, Stern GA: *Pseudomonas* keratitis associated with the use of disposable soft contact lenses, *Arch Ophthalmol* 107:795, 1989.

20. Rabinowitz SM, Pflugfelder SC, Goldberg M: Disposable extended-wear contact lens-related keratitis, *Arch Ophthalmol* 107:1121, 1989.

21. Cohen EJ, Gonzalez C, Leavitt KG, et al: Corneal ulcers associated with contact lenses including experience with disposable lenses, *CLAO* 17:173, 1991.

22. Efron N, Wohl A, Toma NG, et al: *Pseudomonas* corneal ulcers associated with daily wear of disposable hydrogel contact lenses, *Int Cont Lens Clin* 18:46, 1991.

23. Donzis PB, Mondino BJ, Weissman BA et al: Microbial contamination of contact lens care systems, *Am J Ophthalmol* 105(4):325-333, 1987.

24. Hodges EJ, Friedlaender MH, Lee A, et al: Effect of minimal antibiotic treatment on bacterial keratitis, *Cornea* 8(3):188-190, 1989.

25. Weissman BA, Mondino BJ: Ulcerative bacterial keratitis. In Silbert JA (ed): *Anterior Segment Complications of Contact Lens Wear*, New York, 1994, Churchill Livingstone, 247-269.

26. Silbert JA: Microbial infection in contact lens patients. In Harris MG (ed.): *Problems in Optometry: Contact Lenses and Ocular Disease*, Philadelphia, 1990, JB Lippincott, 571-583.

27. Silbert JA: Blepharitis. In Rouse M, Ettinger E (eds): *Clinical Decision Making in Optometry*, 1996, Newton (MA), Butterworth-Heinemann in press.

28. Wilson L: Bacterial corneal ulcers. In Duane TD (ed.): *Clinical Ophthalmology*, Hagerstown, 1976, Harper and Row, Vol 4, Chap 18.

29. Wilson L, Julian A, Ahearn D: The survival and growth of microorganisms in mascara during use, *Am J Ophthalmol* 79:596, 1975.

30. Smolin G: Staphylococcal blepharitis. In Fraunfelder and Roy (eds.): *Current Ocular Therapy*, Philadelphia, 1980, WB Saunders, 435.

31. Ormerod LD, Smith RE: Contact lens-associated microbial keratitis, *Arch Ophthalmol* 104:79-83, 1986.

32. Koidou-Tsiligianni A, Alfonso E, Forster RK: Ulcerative keratitis associated with contact lens wear, *Am J Ophthalmol* 108(1):64-67, 1989.

33. Donnenfield ED, Cohen EJ, Arentsen JJ, et al: Changing trends in contact lens associated corneal ulcers: An overview of 116 cases, *CLAO* 12:145-149, 1986.

34. Cohen EJ, Laibson PR, Arentsen JJ, et al: Corneal ulcers associated with cosmetic extended wear soft lenses, *Ophthalmol* 94:109, 1987.

35. Abbott RL, Abrams MA: Bacterial corneal ulcers. In Duane TD (ed.): *Clinical Ophthalmology*, Philadelphia, 1986, Harper and Row, Vol 4, Chap 18, 1-34.

36. Liesegang TJ: Bacterial and fungal keratitis. In Kaufman HE, Barron BA, McDonald MB, Waltham SR (eds): *The Cornea*, New York, 1988, Churchill Livingstone, 242.

37. Silbert JA: Complications of extended wear. In *Optometry Clinics: Extended Wear*, Norwalk, (Connecticut), 1991, Appleton & Lange, Vol 1, no. 3, 113-114.

38. Moore MB, McCulley JP, Newton C, et al: *Acanthamoeba* keratitis—a growing problem in soft and hard contact lens wearers, *Ophthalmol* 94:1654, 1987.

39. Stehr-Green JK, Bailey TM, Visvesvera GS: The epidemiology of *Acanthamoeba* keratitis in the United States, *Am J Ophthalmol* 107:331, 1989.

40. Ma P, Visvesvera GS, Martinez AJ, et al: *Naegleria* and *Acanthamoeba* infections: review, *Rev Infect Dis* 12:490, 1990.

41. Tarantino N, Anger C, Nelson N, et al: *Acanthamoeba* keratitis and contact lens wear: A review of the literature, *Cont Lens Spectrum* 3(1):57-63, 1988.

42. Koenig SB, Solomon JM, Hyndiuk RA, et al: *Acanthamoeba* keratitis associated with gas-permeable contact lens wear, *Am J Ophthalmol* 102:832, 1987.

43. Kilvington S: *Acanthamoeba* trophozoite and cyst adherence to four types of soft contact lenses and removal by cleaning agents, *Eye* 7:535-538, 1993.

44. White GL, Lundergan MK, Thiese SM, et al: *Acanthamoeba* keratitis: An important consideration when evaluating ocular complaints in contact lens wearers, *J Fam Pract* 27(1):104-107, 1988.

45. Ludwig IH, Meissler DM, Rutherford I, et al: Susceptibility of *Acanthamoeba* to soft contact lens disinfection systems, *Inv Ophthalmol Vis Sci* 27(4):626-628, 1986.

46. Shovlin JP, DePaolis MD, Edmonds SE, et al: *Acanthamoeba* keratitis—contact lenses as a risk factor, *Int Cont Lens Clin* 14:349, 1987.

47. Lindquist TD, Doughman DT, Rubenstein JB, et al: *Acanthamoeba* infected hydrogel contact lenses: Susceptibility to disinfection, ARVO Abstracts, *Inv Ophthalmol Vis Sci* 28:371, 1987.

48. Silvany RE, Wood TS, Bowman RW, et al: The effect of preservatives in contact lens solutions on two species of *Acanthamoeba*, ARVO Abstracts, *Inv Ophthalmol Vis Sci* 28:371, 1987.

49. Penley CA, Willis SW, Sicker SG: Comparative antimicrobial efficacy of soft and rigid gas permeable contact lens solutions against *Acanthamoeba*, *CLAO* 15:257, 1989.

50. Moore MB, McCulley JP, Luckenbach M, et al: *Acanthamoeba* keratitis associated with soft contact lenses, *Am J Ophthalmol* 100(3):396-403, 1985.

51. Florakis GJ, Folberg R, Krachmer JH, et al: Elevated corneal epithelial lines in *Acanthamoeba* keratitis, *Arch Ophthalmol* 106:1202, 1988.

52. Aquavella JV, Shovlin JP, DePaolis MD: Protozoan and fungal keratitis in contact lens wear. In Silbert JA (ed.): *Anterior Segment Complications of Contact Lens Wear*, New York, 1994, Churchill Livingstone, 271-287.

53. Moore MB, McCulley JP, Kaufman HE, et al: Radial keratoneuritis as a presenting sign in *Acanthamoeba* keratitis, *Ophthalmol* 93:1310-1315, 1986.

54. Jones DB: *Acanthamoeba*—the ultimate opportunist?, *Am J Ophthalmol* 103:527-530, 1986.

55. Driebe WT, Stern GA, Epstein RJ, et al: *Acanthamoeba* keratitis: Potential role for topical clotrimazole in combination chemotherapy, *Arch Ophthalmol* 106:1196-1202, 1988.

56. Wilhelmus KR, Robinson NM, Font RA, et al: Fungal keratitis in contact lens wearers, *Am J Ophthalmol* 106:708, 1988.

57. Rosa RH, Miller D, Alfonso EC: The changing spectrum of fungal keratitis in south Florida, *Ophthalmol* 101:1005-1013, 1994.

58. Ando N, Takatori: Fungal flora of the conjunctival sac, *Am J Ophthalmol* 94:67, 1982.

59. Aquavella JV, Shovlin JP, DePaolis MD: Protozoan and fungal keratitis in contact lens wear. In Silbert JA (ed): *Anterior Segment Complications of Contact Lens Wear*, New York, 1994, Churchill Livingstone, 271-287.

60. Chin GN, Hyndiuk RA, Kwasny GP, Schultz RO: Keratomycosis in Wisconsin, *Am J Ophthalmol* 79:121, 1975.

61. Schwartz LK, Loignon LM, Webster RG: Post-traumatic phycomycosis of the anterior segment, *Arch Ophthalmol* 96:860, 1978.

62. Wilson LA, Ahearn DG: Association of fungi with soft contact lenses, *Am J Ophthalmol* 101:434, 1986.

63. Sagan W: Fungal invasion of a soft contact lens, *Arch Ophthalmol* 94:168, 1976.

64. Yamaguchi T, Hubbard A, Fukushima A, et al: Fungus growth on soft contact lenses with different water contents, *CLAO* 10:166, 1984.

65. Penley GA, Llabres C, Wilson LA, Ahearn DG: Efficacy of hydrogen peroxide disinfection systems for soft contact lenses contaminated with fungi, *CLAO* 11:65, 1985.

66. Cakanac CJ: Viral and Chlamydial Infection. In Silbert JA (ed): *Anterior Segment Complications of Contact Lens Wear*, New York, 1994, Churchill Livingstone, 240.

67. Fujikawa LS, Salahuddin SZ, Ablashi D, et al: HTLV-III in the tears of AIDS patients, *Ophthalmol* 93:1479, 1986.
68. DenBeste BP, Hummer J: AIDS: A review and guide for infection control, *J Am Optom Assoc* 57:675-682, 1986.
69. Rajnikant AM, Dean MT, Zaumetzer LE, et al: Viricidal efficacy of various lens cleaning and disinfecting solutions on HIV-1 contaminated contact lenses, *AIDS Res Hum Retroviruses* 7:403, 1991.
70. Centers for Disease Control: Recommendations for preventing possible transmission of human T-lymphotrophic virus type III/lymphadenopathy associated virus from tears, *MMWR* 34:533, 1985.
71. Silbert JA: Ocular inflammation and contact lens wear. In Tomlinson A (ed): *Complications of Contact Lens Wear,* St Louis, 1992, Mosby, 221-235.
72. Silbert JA: The role of inflammation in contact lens wear. In Silbert JA (ed): *Anterior Segment Complications of Contact Lens Wear,* New York, 1994, Churchill Livingstone, 123-141.

2

Dry Eyes and Contact Lens Wear

Charles W. McMonnies

Key Terms

dry eye	surface deposits	biomicroscopy
contact lens	history	

Contact lens wear places additional demands on tear function because of the need to maintain the optical performance of lens surfaces and the health and optical performance of the anterior ocular surface. For most contact lens wearers, these needs are sustained by adequate tear quality, quantity, and blink efficiency so that successful wear is maintained if appropriate lens management strategies are employed. However, for some individuals tear function is less than adequate during contact lens wear and problems develop despite the use of every resource to prevent them. For individual cases, it is not always known whether there is reduced tear function before lens wear or whether a reduction in tear quality, quantity, and blink efficiency during lens wear has led to inferior contact lens performance.

For example, contact lens wear has been associated with increased mucus production,[1] reduced blink efficiency,[2] 3-9 o'clock epithelial stain,[3] reduced tear break-up time,[4] increased tear evaporation,[5] and increased lysozyme and lactoferrin concentration.[6] Some of the physical mechanisms whereby a contact lens interferes with the tear film and its function have been described.[3] Studies that measured water loss from hydrogel lenses on the eye[5-8] indicated a potential for problems related to the loss of hydration. These problems include reduced oxygen transmission, tightening of fit, power change, reduced vision, increased surface deposits, increased lens awareness, and increased risk of infection. Increased adherence of silicone lenses to the eye because of fluid loss through evaporation has been reported.[9]

The development of a dry eye condition as a consequence of contact lens wear has been reported[10] even in cases that present as having normal tears before fitting. It is probable that dry eye patients are susceptible to adverse reactions to contact lens solution preservatives when reduced tear volume or flow results in greater concentrations of preservative being in contact with the tissues for longer periods. Dry eye tissue may be less protected and less able to withstand the toxic or sensitizing potential of solution preservatives. Reduced tear function that pre-exists contact lens wear could be exacerbated when contact lenses are worn. Thus marginal tear deficiencies associated with mild symptoms and signs may become significant when contact lenses are worn. A questionnaire that examined for dry eye symptoms was completed by 500 patients who presented for refractive error correction, and it was found that contact lens wearers reported symptoms more frequently than nonwearers ($p < .0001$) and that soft lens wearers reported symptoms more frequently than hard lens wearers ($p < .01$).[11]

CLINICAL PEARL

Marginal tear deficiencies associated with mild symptoms and signs may become significant when contact lenses are worn.

The symptom options offered in the questionnaire were soreness, scratchiness, dryness, grittiness, and burning. When three or more nominal options are offered in a questionnaire, there is the possibility of a primacy effect,[12] in which respondents rank the choices for frequency of use in the exact order of their sequence of presentation. In the analysis of responses from nonwearers a primacy effect was found[11] that might indicate a reduced capacity to discriminate among descriptive options when symptoms are less severe.[12]

The choice of words to describe symptoms is not completely understood. In the absence of a specific ocular sensory basis for symptom descriptions, a report of one or more of the options may be based on an individual's impression of an ocular sensation matching a similar sensation elsewhere in the body (for example, a parched throat that may feel dry, sore, scratchy, or burning). Table 2-1 shows the frequency with which the symptom options were used by nonwearers, soft lens wearers, and hard lens wearers. Interestingly, despite

TABLE 2-1

Frequency of Use of Symptom Descriptions for Nonwearers and Contact Lens Wearers

Symptom Description	Percentage of use		
	NW[*]	SCL[†]	HCL[‡]
Soreness	37	24	21
Scratchiness	21	14	14
Grittiness	15	18	24
Burning	14	13	9
Dryness	12	32	31

NW, nonwearer; *SCL*, soft lens wearer; *HCL*, hard (rigid) lens wearer.
[*]n = 177; [†]n = 163; [‡]n = 160.

the possible influence of a primacy effect, the least common option for nonwearers (dryness) is the most common option chosen by both groups of contact lens wearers.

Tear function can be altered by contact lens wear, but also is burdened by the need to maintain a nondesquamating contact lens surface capable of accumulating tear residues and showing reduced tear break-up time. It may therefore be more appropriate to describe the symptoms of lens wearers as dry lens symptoms rather than dry eye symptoms.

Prevalence

The prevalence of keratoconjunctivitis sicca (KCS) is unknown for patients who present for contact lens fitting. In a review of estimates of the prevalence of KCS in ophthalmological practice, it was concluded that de Roetth's estimate of 1 patient in 620 was probably valid.[13] The prevalence would be expected to vary depending on the type of practice and the practitioner's interest in the disease. For patients who present for correction of refractive errors with contact lenses, the prevalence of KCS is likely to be considerably less than that found in ophthalmological practice. The high prevalence of symptoms among contact lens wearers suggests that lens wear is a provocative test for tear function, causing marginal or incipient tear dysfunction to become apparent.

Consequences

The principal consequence of reduced tear function is contact lens surface degradation, including excess deposition of tear residues. When tear fluid is collected, placed on a microscope cover slip, and

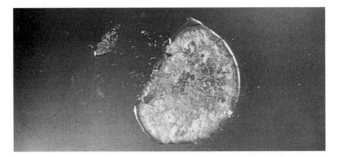

FIGURE 2-1 A precipitate of solid tear components formed by allowing a tear sample to dry on a microscope cover slip, illustrating the potential for tear components to deposit on contact lens surfaces.

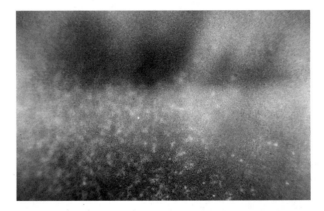

FIGURE 2-2 A clearly demarcated zone of corneal epitheliopathy observed in a wearer of toric soft lenses. The "prow line" associated with incomplete blinking separates desiccated and healthy epithelium.

allowed to dry, an opaque residue results (Figure 2-1). The tendency for surface deposits to form on the front contact lens surface, far in excess to those that form on the back surface, suggests that precipitation of solid tear matter is a principal mechanism for deposition. The mechanism is demonstrated in nonrotating lenses used to correct astigmatism. If an incomplete blink mechanism fails to maintain front surface wetness, precipitates concentrate on the lower (exposed) part of the nonrotating lens front surface (Figures 2-2 and 2-3). Clinicians have long recognized the association of incomplete blinking, lens surface drying, and surface deposits.[14] Contact lenses may reduce blink efficiency[15] and cause tear deficiency. Incomplete blinking has been associated with an increased rate of dehydration in the lower

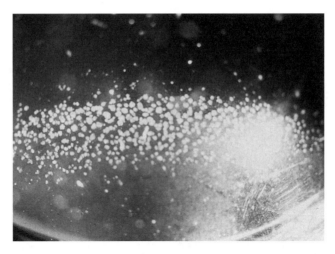

FIGURE 2-3 Surface deposit formed on a toric (nonrotating) soft lens and concentrated in the exposed lens area where incomplete blinking exaggerates precipitation of solid tear components.

part of soft lenses, exposure stain, surface deposits, and dry eye symptoms.[16] These effects are apparent in nonrotating (prism ballast/truncated/toric) lenses (hard or soft) when surface deposits develop more obviously in the lens' exposed area (see Figures 2-2 and 2-3).

At one extreme of the range of patient types, adequate tear quantity, quality, and blink efficiency allow wearers to experience few problems with lens soilage. For patients at the other extreme of the range, a maximum effort in lens maintenance is insufficient to prevent rapid precipitation of deposits.

In a detailed analysis of 600 aftercare visits the most common area of remedial/management/prophylactic action (one third of the total) was concerned with control of surface deposits.[17] Ideally, the patient at risk for surface deposits and other tear–deficiency-related problems could be identified before fitting, and appropriate prescribing and prophylactic management recommendations could be employed so that wearing problems are reduced or avoided. The principal clinical challenge is to employ appropriate screening and diagnostic methods to detect patients at risk for tear–deficiency-related problems. The task is difficult because prospective contact lens wearers at risk for problems are much more likely to manifest marginal tear deficiency than established dry eye pathology. Because the majority (more than 90%) of people presenting for contact lens fitting for refractive error correction appear to have normal tear function,[11] the question arises as to how much examination time should be allowed for effective examination of tear function in routine contact lens practice.

Screening for Tear Deficiency

Screening for and diagnosis of tear function anomalies are frequently difficult, especially in marginal cases. Signs do not always correlate with symptoms and even in well-established cases different signs are found across the range of tear deficiency states. A further complication derives from other diseases that have signs and symptoms in common with tear deficiency. The most commonly cited condition associated with tear deficiency is chronic blepharoconjunctivitis.[18-20] Other conditions that may have signs and symptoms in common with dry eye include rosacea keratoconjunctivitis,[21] allergic conjunctivitis,[20] and lower lid laxity.[22] In many clinical situations history taking provides a high diagnostic potential.[23] However, in the case of tear deficiency diagnosis the clinician has the complex task of determining the relative significance of primary and secondary (provoked) symptoms and a range of ocular and systemic factors that may only sometimes be associated with a dry eye. For example, a history of rheumatoid arthritis is usually unrelated to a dry eye state but can be an important component in the recognition of Sjögren's syndrome. It is useful to collect a wide range of information even though some of it may only occasionally be relevant to a tear deficiency diagnosis. Because the collection of history information by direct interrogation is time consuming, a compromise solution is to use a questionnaire that can be completed outside the consulting room with supervision from an assistant. The potential disadvantage of this approach is that responses may have reduced validity if the questions are not well understood.

An appropriate questionnaire should examine for symptoms that occur without provocation (primary symptoms) and symptoms that occur under provocative conditions (secondary symptoms). Provocative conditions include cigarette smoke, smog, air conditioning, central heating, alcohol, water when swimming, and parasympatholytic or sympatholytic drugs that decrease tear production. The questionnaire should examine for connective tissue disease such as rheumatoid arthritis, and sicca conditions in nonocular mucous membranes such as dry mouth (xerostomia) to indicate the risk for Sjögren's syndrome. Other conditions that may be associated with tear deficiency that should be examined for include thyroid abnormality, nocturnal lagophthalmos, and recurrent corneal erosion, as a means of estimating the risk of corneal exposure syndrome during contact lens wear. The questionnaire should determine if previous treatment has been prescribed for tear deficiency. Self-medication is not as significant as prescribed treatment.

It has been shown that a questionnaire based on these areas of inquiry[24] is capable of successfully discriminating between normal subjects and sicca subjects.[11] The questionnaire responses for age and

sex matched samples of sicca syndrome patients, and patients presenting for refractive error correction were compared using discriminant
analysis. A correct classification was found for 62 of 63 sicca subjects
and for 36 of 37 normal subjects, representing 98% sensitivity and 97%
specificity. An equivocal classification that warranted supplementary
diagnostic procedures was indicated for 5% of subjects. A referent
level of 5% to be given additional diagnostic procedures yields a
sensitivity of 100%. These results indicate that the questionnaire will
obviate the need for supplementary ocular sicca examination for 95%
of patients presenting for refractive error correction.

CLINICAL PEARL

*It has been shown that a questionnaire based on these areas of inquiry is
capable of successfully discriminating between normal subjects and sicca
subjects.*

However, patients presenting for contact lens fitting have a risk of
increased tear deficiency symptoms[11] and signs.[17]

Women More Than 45 Years Old

Established tear deficiency conditions are more common in postmeno-
pausal women,[18] but their prevalence among contact lens patients is
low.[11] No evidence exists that female contact lens patients more than
45 years old are at greater risk for developing tear deficiency problems
when contact lenses are worn. Surprisingly, some of the evidence is to
the contrary. An analysis of symptoms related to tear deficiency among
normal subjects[25] indicated a reduction in the reporting of primary
symptoms as age increases. Reports of soreness ($p < .01$) and burning
($p < .003$) reduced with age, as did the frequency of primary symptoms
($p < .05$). The reduction in primary symptom reporting found among
normal patients as age increases may have several explanations, including reduced corneal sensitivity, the acceptance of chronic symptoms as normal, and an associated tendency to understate or not report
them. Ocular symptoms may be considered mild when compared to
nonocular symptoms that develop with increasing age.

Biomicroscopy

Marginal tear deficiency conditions that are usually encountered in
contact lens practice are unlikely to be associated with the obvious
signs found in well-established tear deficiency pathology. Nevertheless, because biomicroscopic evaluation is a routine part of contact

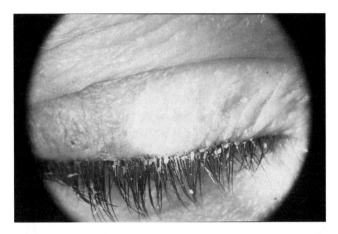

FIGURE 2-4 Blepharitis condition that should be treated and brought under control before contact lens wear is initiated. The condition should then be managed carefully to prevent acute episodes during lens wear so that symptoms (especially those that mimic tear deficiency) can be avoided or minimized.

lens examinations, when tear deficiency is suspected on the basis of symptoms and related provocative or systemic conditions, the diagnostic potential for biomicroscopy should be fully realized. It is important to follow an appropriate sequence of biomicroscopic observations to ensure maximum validity and reliability of results. For example, the insertion of trial lenses, lid eversion, instillation of fluorescein or rose bengal, or any other invasive procedure can obliterate signs of tear deficiency and should not be employed until preliminary observations are completed.

A prime concern in a tear deficiency biomicroscopic sequence is to examine for and differentially diagnose conditions that mimic tear deficiency symptoms. Examination of the skin and adnexa may indicate a rosacea condition, lower lid laxity, lid redness, or the presence of blepharitis scales (Figure 2-4). Absolute differential diagnosis between tear deficiency and external eye diseases that can cause the same symptoms is not always possible or necessary. It is prudent to allow the possibility that tear deficiency and external eye conditions can be present together and that the most effective management may require treatment of both conditions.

Frequently, differential diagnosis cannot be made with confidence, especially when a combination of mild to moderate conditions is present. In these cases the syndrome of mild to moderate, mostly chronic conditions gives a clinical picture of chronically red and irritated eyes that may be associated with a history of allergy or other conditions with symptoms similar to tear deficiency. These eyes can be described as "reactive" because of their hypersensitivity to every-

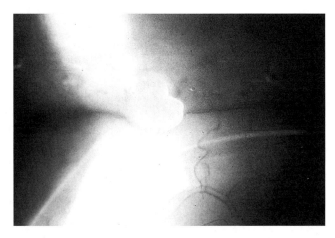

FIGURE 2-5 A solid plug of waxy sebum extruding from a meibomian gland orifice. Meibomian gland dysfunction needs to be controlled to improve tear quality and reduce tear deficiency symptoms.

day stimuli such as wind, dust, smoke, smog, glare, lack of sleep, eyestrain, alcohol, air conditioning, and central heating.[26] They may more easily show a reduced tear function side effect of medication [24] and may react adversely to contact lens wear, resulting in greater hyperemia and increased surface deposits.

For example, the clinical spectrum of chronic blepharitis includes infection with *Staphylococcus aureus* alone or in combination with seborrheic dermatitis or acne rosacea (with or without associated excess meibomian gland secretions or inflammation). In a study of these conditions, keratoconjunctivitis sicca was a frequent finding.[27]

After the examination of skin, adnexa, and lids, the lid margins and meibomian gland orifices should be examined. Signs of meibomian gland dysfunction include excessive oiliness, inspissated waxy sebum plugging of orifices (Figure 2-5), localized swelling and redness, and the formation of froth or foam along the lid margin and at the canthi. Lid eversion is necessary to detect an internal hordeolum or a chalazion that has broken through to the conjunctival surface. However, eversion negates the validity of other findings by stimulating reflex tears and increasing the quantity of tear debris visible over the corneal surface. For this reason, lid eversion should be delayed until other invasive procedures such as the instillation of stains are performed.

The next step is an examination of the regularity of lid margins, because tear distribution anomalies (for example, dry spots and short tear break-up time) may result from lid margin and tear distribution irregularities.

Abnormalities in lacrimal drainage may be indicated by anomalies of punctal position or patency. Examination of the marginal tear prism or meniscus is not a reliable guide to tear volume.[28] Adequate tear volume should be evident from a complete tear prism appearance (full height). However, tear prism height may vary with poor lid-globe apposition (ectropion will reduce tear prism height, for example), variations in tear surface tension, the presence of bulbar conjunctival folds, momentary reflex tearing induced by the examination, or with other factors unrelated to tear volume. Notwithstanding this observation's unreliability, reduced tear prism height is a clue to reduced tear volume when there is no other apparent cause.

The presence of large amounts of tear debris suggests reduced tear volume or flow. Normal desquamated epithelium may accumulate and mucin concentration (including the formation of viscous mucin threads) may provide evidence of reduced tear volume or flow. Observation of corneal specular reflection during three or four normal blinks will disclose tear debris, but care should be taken to rule out the possibility of excess tear debris caused by increased mucin production (as with any conjunctival inflammation, for example) or by a previous lid eversion procedure.

The specular reflection from the bulbar conjunctiva is normally bright and appears wet, but tear deficiency leads to a dull conjunctival specular reflex that shows a granular and relatively dry appearance.

Examination of the corneal conjunctival reflex using high magnification may disclose signs of excess lipid such as colored interference patterns, or signs of an incomplete lipid layer dispersion that causes the normal regular reflex to show lenses of lipid or a crumpled, textured, uneven appearance.[29] It is important to discriminate between disturbances to the reflex from debris that breaks through the tear layer surface and irregularities in the lipid layer's continuity, which does not have a three-dimensional aspect.

To ensure the validity of observations made to this point in the biomicroscopic sequence, all invasive procedures should have been avoided. Potentially invasive procedures include the instillation of stains, lid eversion (even the lower lid, but especially the upper lid), manipulation of swollen painful lids, and attempts to express inspissated plugs from meibomian gland orifices. For photophobic patients even the biomicroscope illumination source can provoke lacrimation.

Rose bengal stains devitalized cells and precipitated mucin, both of which are abundant in established keratoconjunctivitis sicca. Fluorescein stain may be found in many conditions (including *Staphylococcus* infection, rosacea, and allergy) that requires differential diagnosis from tear deficiency, and serves to prompt closer examination with rose bengal. Mucous strands within the tear film also are more clearly disclosed by fluorescein stain. Notwithstanding rose bengal's diagnostic value in established tear deficiency pathology, it is rarely used for routine screening of contact lens patients.[30] This form of examination can be omitted and used only as a supplementary test if tear deficiency is suggested by fluorescein stain or other findings. If rose bengal stain is used for all screening examinations, it can most conveniently be added to a fluorescein strip and instilled in combination with fluorescein.

The first blinks following fluorescein instillation allow assessment of tear distribution, aid detection of dry spots associated with epitheliopathy (fixed location and formed almost instantaneously), and provide evidence of tear instability via random areas of tear break-up that form within the normal interblink period. Tear instability indicated by tear break-up within a normal interblink period (around 5 or 6 seconds) can be a sign of mucin deficiency, lipid abnormality, or impaired lid function. Measuring tear break-up time with a stopwatch after asking the patient to avoid blinking is a provocative test, but findings of less than 10 seconds are abnormal. To approach reasonably reliable results, this form of provocative testing needs to be repeated several times, with the increasing likelihood of reflex tearing diluting the stain and spoiling observations as the patient attempts to avoid blinking. For these reasons, this provocative test can be omitted and the absence of tear break-up within normal interblink periods can be a guide to satisfactory tear stability.

A number of useful observations can be made following the instillation of stains. For example, when aqueous deficiency is present the dilution of fluorescein is limited and hypofluorescence can be observed. Confirmation of reduced tear bulk occurs when a dull fluorescence (sometimes a dull orange color) is seen under ultraviolet examination. Care must be taken to ensure that hypofluorescence is not caused by incomplete instillation or rapid stain dilution (washout) following reflex tearing stimulated by instillation.

If the opposite occurs and the elimination of fluorescein is delayed, there can be suspicion of reduced tear bulk or turnover. If a stopwatch is started at the time of fluorescein instillation, an ultraviolet examination after 5 minutes may disclose significant retained tear prism fluorescence. Measurement of tear volume and tear flow[31,32] indicates that complete tear exchange normally occurs in about 5 minutes. Although this period may be different after instillation of stain, all that is required is the discrimination between the normal reading of almost complete elimination of stain after 5 minutes and the suspicious finding of significant residual fluorescence after 5 minutes. This simple observation (abstracted from the Norn streak dilution test) is completed after biomicroscopy and also indicates if irrigation is needed before the insertion of soft trial lenses.

Delayed fluorescein elimination also may be caused by impaired lacrimal drainage and may warrant an investigation of the drainage system's patency.

Staining of the most exposed lower area of cornea and conjunctiva can indicate incomplete or infrequent blinking, exophthalmos, or nocturnal lagophthalmos. When any of these conditions are present to a mild degree, exposure stain can be exacerbated during visual tasks involving intense visual effort that reduces blink completeness or frequency. Exposure stain may heal during the morning and not be evident at an afternoon examination. The presence of a Hudson-Stahli line, however, suggests chronic epithelial damage[33]; the refractile changes associated with epithelial basement membrane dystrophy also may indicate the potential for poor epithelial attachment.

Summary

Biomicroscopy is an art as well as a science. Most observations are difficult to quantify and, in relation to signs of tear deficiency, many findings are transient or variable. Fortunately, many clues aid diagnosis. For prospective contact lens patients, marginal tear deficiency is encountered much more frequently than established tear deficiency pathology, and usually a tentative diagnosis is an appropriate basis for conservative prescribing and management decisions. The diagnosis of marginal tear deficiency is stronger or weaker depending on the symptoms' intensity and frequency, the presence of associated factors derived from a comprehensive questionnaire, and the number and severity of positive signs encountered during a biomicroscopic examination.

The following recommended biomicroscopy sequence was described earlier:

1. Examine for conditions that mimic tear deficiency symptoms.
2. Evaluate regularity of lid margins, tear prism height, and lid apposition.
3. Estimate the brightness of the specular reflex from the conjunctiva and cornea, and determine the levels of the precorneal tear debris.
4. Investigate the lipid layer's integrity.
5. Introduce stains and examine for hypofluorescence, tear instability, adequacy of tear spreading, incomplete blinking, conjunctival and corneal exposure, and delayed elimination of stain.

Special Tests

For the vast majority of contact lens patients, a comprehensive dry eye history and a biomicroscopy examination for signs of tear deficiency are adequate screening procedures. A history questionnaire completed outside the consulting room and routine biomicroscopy with an emphasis on the detection of signs of dry eye can be time efficient for the practitioner. Additional tests, however, are not time efficient.

For example, a Schirmer's tear test will prevent other examination procedures for at least 6 minutes. Moreover, the usefulness of Schirmer's tests is limited in contact lens practice when marginal tear deficiency, rather than established dry eye pathology, is encountered. Schirmer's testing without anesthesia (Schirmer I) has been found useful in patients with Sjögren's syndrome.[34] However, Schirmer's testing is unreliable in normal subjects,[35,36] and Schirmer's testing with local anesthesia (Schirmer II) has been found unreliable because reflex tearing is not always completely suppressed.[37,38] Special tests involving assays of tear components to indicate tear deficiency are not time efficient for routine contact lens patient screening. For example, lysozyme assays are cumbersome to perform and require a laboratory capable of completing them on a routine basis.[39]

When evidence suggests a tear deficiency condition beyond a marginal stage, which is rare for routine contact lens practice, additional tests such as the Schirmer's test or the cotton thread test[40] can be used.

However, should advanced tear deficiency be diagnosed, appropriate management will be to advise against contact lens wear. For prospective wearers diagnosed as having marginal tear deficiency, a fitting can proceed, but the sooner appropriate conservative management is introduced the more successful can be the final outcome.

A diagnosis of tear deficiency or reactive eye conditions such as blepharitis before fitting contact lenses provides an opportunity for problems to be avoided or reduced. The patient should be told that success with contact lenses depends on his or her ability to avoid excess wear. Limited daily wear of 10 to 12 hours per day is an appropriate initial goal. Extended wear is contraindicated. Disposable lenses can be indicated on a daily-wear basis.

Greater emphasis than normal is required in establishing patient compliance with wearing and maintenance instructions. The patient who is advised from the outset that lens wear should be avoided during provocative circumstances such as long periods of study, is easier to manage than one who initially establishes a 16- or 17-hour-per day habit and then needs to reduce wear when signs of tear deficiency develop. In all cases contact lens wear proves or disproves the significance of tear deficiency for individual patients.

Contact lens wear is a provocative test for tear deficiency. When compliance with maintenance instructions is established, the finding at aftercare examinations of greater than expected surface deposits indicates tear deficiency. Sometimes, after only 2 weeks of use lenses will show abnormal surface deposition, prompting reaffirmation of the advice given at the prescribing visit and additional advice concerning management.

Apart from surface deposition, aftercare visits may disclose other signs of tear deficiency. Lenses that do not wet properly may indicate contamination of tears with excess lipid production. Excess debris, especially fine emulsified froth trapped under lenses, is another clue to tear deficiency.

Superficial punctate corneal epitheliopathy can indicate tear deficiency. For example, staining with fluorescein may indicate peripheral exposure epithelial desiccation (3-9 or 4-8 o'clock stain) in rigid lens wearers or inferior corneal exposure stain in soft lens wearers (see Figure 2-2), especially those wearing toric lenses.[16] These signs of contact–lens-provoked tear deficiency may be complicated by poor quality lens material, manufacturing, or fitting, and are considered in a discussion of management procedures in the next section.

Recognizing Tear Deficiency When Contact Lenses Are Worn

Tear function in contact lens wear is so critically important that tear deficiency can become apparent within weeks of using new lenses. Even marginal tear deficiencies that are difficult to diagnose before lens wear may be clearly evident after lens wear. As stated earlier, lens wear is a provocative test for tear deficiency. The time taken for tear deficiency to become evident is a fairly reliable guide to the degree of the problem, although adverse wear conditions that place additional demands on tear function will hasten the onset of signs and symptoms. In fact, when conditions are particularly demanding even normal tear function may be unable to sustain contact lens wear. Factors that increase demand on tear function include dry atmospheric conditions, wind, high temperatures, and vision tasks that inhibit the frequency and completeness of blinking. Under these conditions, tear deficiency can be classified as conditional because normal contact lens performance is experienced when adverse wear conditions change or can be avoided.

Symptoms of Tear Deficiency When Contact Lenses Are Worn

Contact lens wearers and nonwearers use similar words to describe symptoms of tear deficiency.[30] Soreness, scratchiness, dryness, grittiness, and burning are all commonly used terms, with dryness being the most common symptom and burning the least (see Table 2-1). These symptoms may not necessarily be caused by tear deficiency. Damaged, ill-fitting, or poorly manufactured lenses may cause grittiness, scratchiness, or soreness. Other symptom descriptions used by contact lens wearers may be less associated with tear deficiency. Stinging may be associated with mild to moderate chemical trauma, and itchiness may be associated with allergic responses. However, no one symptom is unique to tear deficiency, and reports of symptoms necessitate a careful history and biomicroscopic examination to detect whether external eye conditions, contact lens fit, or manufacturing quality are responsible. Frequently it is not possible to differentially diagnose a particular cause of symptoms, and several management strategies may be appropriate.

Signs of Tear Deficiency When Contact Lenses Are Worn

Tear deficiency leads to disturbance in contact lens wetness with associated surface degradation that causes reduced optical performance and comfort. Moreover, the possibility exists of adverse tissue changes. Although adequately cleaned and wetted before insertion, any lens may dry out on the eye. Wetness needs to be maintained by tears in combination with efficient blinking. In some cases of lipid tear contamination the loss of wetness can occur within a few minutes, rendering the prelens tear layer unstable. Under these circumstances tear break-up can rapidly occur during normal interblink intervals. If lenses are clean and wet at insertion, deposit formation during wear is a measure of tear deficiency.[41] Deposits on the exposed (inferior) lens surface indicate incomplete blink patterns and will be particularly apparent on nonrotating lenses. Incomplete blink patterns may create annular ("dinner plate pattern") deposits on rotating lenses and result in the entire front surface periphery progressively being located at the inferior position where exposure occurs. As in the case of symptoms, signs of contact–lens-related tear deficiency may at least partly be caused by factors other than tear-related deficiency. Before attributing surface deposits to tear deficiency, it is necessary to confirm the patient's compliance with maintenance procedures. Surface deposits may be a function of inferior manufacturing technique, causing poorly polished lens surfaces to be difficult to wet and easy to soil. Apart from tear deficiency, the presence of significant surface deposits at aftercare visits warrants a careful differential diagnosis among all other possible contributing factors. Frequently, many causes will be suspected or identified, requiring a comprehensive approach to management.

Tissue Changes from Tear Deficiency When Contact Lenses Are Worn

Tissue changes from tear deficiency in contact lens wear can show characteristic epitheliopathy for different lens types. Peripheral exposure fluorescein stain (3-9 o'clock or 4-8 o'clock stain) is a frequent finding with rigid lenses. Sometimes toric soft lenses are associated with epitheliopathy limited to the exposed inferior corneal region (see Figure 2-2). Any type of lens can be associated with diffuse widespread stain if soiled lenses are worn.

Epitheliopathy occurs under a wide variety of conditions unrelated to tear deficiency or contact lens wear, and requires careful differential diagnosis so that all possible causes can be considered when management decisions are made.

Prevention, Remediation, and Management of Contact–Lens-Related Tear Deficiency

Contact lens wear can be successfully sustained despite marginal tear deficiency conditions. However, the routine recommendation of tear supplements without consideration of other methods of relieving symptoms is poor clinical practice. Many patients report dissatisfaction with tear supplement use because tear deficiency symptoms return quickly after a short period of relief. In many of these cases insufficient effort is made to identify the coexistence of multiple features of tear deficiency or to recognize conditions that mimic tear deficiency signs and symptoms. A comprehensive approach to the identification of various causes and subsequent broad-range management procedures may give significant improvement without supplements.

CLINICAL PEARL

The routine recommendation of tear supplements without consideration of other methods of relieving symptoms is poor clinical practice.

Although many of the principles of managing established dry eye conditions can be adapted to the management of contact–lens-induced tear deficiency, contact lenses are contraindicated for established pathological dry eye conditions.[42-43] The foreign body status of contact lenses increases the degree of tear deficiency and the risk of significant tissue damage and infection. It is useful to regard contact–lens-induced tear deficiency as a dry lens problem rather than a dry eye problem. For patients at risk for problems, prescribing decisions and early management are important. Lens choices may influence final outcomes, but the evidence concerning the relative advantages of high and low water content soft lenses does not clearly indicate which is superior in individual cases. Very thin low water content soft lenses can be associated with increased epithelial abrasion and high water content soft lenses can soil more readily, but exceptions to these generalities will be found. Some patients may have greater success in rigid lenses, although gas-permeable rigid lenses can sometimes develop significant surface deposits. The surface quality achieved during manufacture may be more important than material choice. Insufficient knowledge exists on which to make broad generalizations about lens design and material choice when managing tear deficiency problems. It is nevertheless useful to consider a change in lens design or material when seeking improvements for individual patients.

When contact–lens-induced tear deficiency results from or is complicated by medications that have the potential to alter tear function, management procedures may be needed only during periods of medication, or may need to be intensified during such periods. Patients must understand the possible relationship between their medication and their contact lens performance. Contact lens wearers with such awareness are capable of anticipating problems, modifying lens use, and reducing wearing time for the duration of the use of the suspected medication. Similarly, for some people alcohol consumption is associated with temporary reduction in tear function the day after consumption. Identification of this mechanism can contribute to reduction in symptoms through better management of wearing times.

Abstinence from contact lens wear may be needed to show the contribution of external eye conditions that mimic tear deficiency symptoms or signs. Occasionally, a chronic allergic condition can be identified and treated with sensitization to cosmetics or contact lens maintenance products used over long periods. Frequently, contact–lens-induced tear deficiency can be complicated by external eye conditions that require treatment for maximal relief of signs and symptoms. In fact, sometimes the management of an external eye condition such as blepharitis is the most important component in achieving symptomatic relief.

Severe forms of blepharitis contraindicate contact lens wear, and new fittings should be postponed until appropriate medical treatment has brought the condition under control.[43] There remains the need to treat blepharitis conditions during contact lens wear so that they are kept under control; management should include lid hygiene and treatment for seborrhea when appropriate. Hot compresses should be recommended to remove blepharitis crusts from lashes and promote conditions less conducive to the growth and activity of resident *Staphylococcus* bacteria. A clean washcloth can be brought to a steaming hot condition by running it under hot water and wringing it out. The face cloth should be as hot as the hands are able to withstand comfortably and used to gently massage the lashes and lid margins to free them from crusts, accumulated secretions, dust, and foreign matter that collects on lashes as a normal part of their protective function. This procedure performed night and morning will increase resistance to outbreaks of blepharitis. Patients with seborrhea may need to be advised about appropriate control measures, because seborrhea scales can fall from the hair and eyebrows and be a major source of lash contamination. These patients may need advice regarding the regular use of medicated shampoo and the need to wash their scalps and hair (including eyebrows), which can be an unsuspected and direct source of lash-contaminating scales.

Meibomian gland dysfunction also should be treated as a means of relieving contact–lens-related tear deficiency.[44] When meibomian gland ducts become plugged, they may require expression by applying pressure through the lid against a cotton tip applicator held against the palpebral conjunctiva. Home therapy includes hot compresses using a hot washcloth as described earlier, but emphasizing lid massage. The combination of heat and massage will help restore and maintain duct patency and establish satisfactory lid hygiene. A nonirritant shampoo can be used with a cotton tip applicator to clear the lid margin of waxy sebum secretions that accumulate at the gland orifice.[44]

Marginal tear deficiency conditions are more likely to be associated with symptoms under provocative environmental conditions. Dry, hot, or windy climates, air conditioning, central heating, cigarette smoke, and smog can all be provocative factors that warrant consideration in efforts to maintain tear function during contact lens wear. Similarly, swimmers sometimes find their marginal tear deficiency condition exacerbated after swimming. The tears cannot adequately recover from the irritation and dilution that occurs while swimming, and contact lens wear is adversely affected. Although patients usually are able to identify these problems, it is sometimes necessary to promote understanding and acceptance that these factors can contribute to contact–lens-related tear deficiency problems and that it is necessary to avoid or compensate for them with protection or with symptom-relieving treatment.

Provocative environmental conditions are more likely to be adversely significant if corneal exposure results from infrequent or incomplete blinking. Contact lens wear may reduce blink efficiency. Tasks that require intense visual concentration also will reduce blink efficiency. Touch typing, working with video display terminals, and inspection operations on production lines are all vision tasks involving intense concentration that can lead to reduced blink frequency and completeness. In some cases of contact–lens-related tear deficiency, improving blink efficiency is critical in relieving signs and symptoms.[15,45] With improved blink efficiency, surface deposition is reduced, tear circulation is promoted, lens movement and centering are enhanced, and vision performance is increased. The difficult task is to motivate the patient to take the time and make the necessary effort to improve blink efficiency. In most cases the patient would prefer that the resolution of his or her symptoms be achieved with some form of lens or maintenance system modification. Nevertheless, the time taken to explain how blink inefficiency causes symptoms and signs is the most important aspect of management. Having the patient understand the problem is the key to motivating him or her to become actively involved in achieving improvement. Photographs and printed information that display and describe blink phenomena are essential to this cause. Printed information should include specific instructions regarding methods used in practicing complete blinking (see Appendix 2-1).[46] An additional set of instructions is included (see Appendix 2-2)[47] to provide alternative ideas for helping the patient improve blink efficiency.

CLINICAL PEARL

With improved blink efficiency, surface deposition is reduced, tear circulation is promoted, lens movement and centering are enhanced, and vision performance is increased.

Improving blink efficiency is an important aspect of attempts to relieve peripheral corneal exposure desiccation (3-9 o'clock and 4-8 o'clock stain). If, as is suspected, this epitheliopathy results from deficient lid massage, improvement will occur if blink efficiency is improved. In particular, when the epithelial desiccation is found at 4-8 o'clock (lid closure stain)[45] in association with inferior lens location caused by incomplete blinks, improved blink efficiency will give better lens centration and reduce epithelial exposure. Other means of remediating peripheral corneal exposure desiccation include fit improvements to reduce edge thickness and clearance and to aid better lens centration. Changes in overall lens diameter may help. Improvement may be found by increasing lens wettability (through better material or maintenance) and giving attention to all other aspects of tear deficiency management. Difficult cases will lead to peripheral scarring and necessitate reduction in wearing time, although a change to soft lenses is often a preferred option.

For any patient with tear–deficiency-related contact lens signs and symptoms, a reduction in wearing time can be a crucial element in a complete remedial strategy. Contact lens wearers do not need to continue wear until bedtime when circumstances permit earlier removal. Lenses that accumulate problem surface deposits during wear should be cleaned and rehydrated or rewetted before evening wear if a late night is expected. However, if the patient is at home without a need to continue lens wear, problems will be greatly reduced if he or she changes to spectacles. A few hours less wear means an increased period in which to recover from adverse responses. The extra recovery time during waking hours has the advantages associated with blinking and increased oxygen availability for recovery from hypoxia and tissue change when compared to recovery time during sleep. A few hours' reduction in wear carries a double bonus—not only extra waking time for recovery but also fewer surface deposits, less epitheliopathy, and less hypoxia from which to recover.

All efforts should be made to control surface deposits. Aftercare visits should include careful assessment of the patient's compliance with maintenance instructions; efforts should be intensified where possible. Lenses should be replaced more frequently; daily wear disposable lenses or frequent replacement lenses are often the answer to intractable deposit problems.

The tear deficiency problems experienced by contact lens wearers can present a conflict in choosing the most appropriate tear supplement. A potential for conflict exists between the therapeutic needs of the tissue surfaces and the need to maintain or re-establish the lens surface's quality. Some products are formulated for nonwearers. For example, in an aqueous deficient eye the ocular surface may benefit most from a non-viscous aqueous bulk replacement, whereas the surface of a lens worn on that eye may require a drop containing a viscous adsorptive polymer with a potential to enhance the lens surface's wettability.

Several features of tear supplement formulas may influence the results obtained (for example, whether or not preservatives are included, and the tonicity, buffering, and pH of the solution all can be important determinants of patient response). Adverse reactions to preservatives in tear supplements may occur frequently in contact lens wearers whose tear function and ocular surface integrity are reduced by lens wear. Unit dose nonpreserved tear supplements can be useful in avoiding these reactions. Patients can dismiss certain products because they feel uncomfortable on insertion or because vision is blurred for a few minutes after insertion. These conflicts of choice and problems in use cannot be resolved without comparative trials, and patients often benefit most by using a different product for each eye so that the most beneficial can be identified. Inappropriate tear supplement recommendations that give short-term benefit may lead to overuse and the risk of too frequent tear dilution that causes symptoms rather than gives relief. Tear supplements play a vital role in the management of contact–lens-related tear deficiency, but it is poor clinical practice to prescribe them routinely, because they may not be needed if full attention is given to other means of management described earlier in this chapter.

Punctal occlusion may reduce dryness symptoms in contact lens wearers who do not respond to other procedures or for whom tear supplement application is inconvenient. The procedure is indicated for eyes with reduced aqueous production.[48] Patients with adequate aqueous production who suffer from dry lens symptoms caused by unwettable or soiled lens surfaces are unlikely to benefit from punctal occlusion. They are more likely to be annoyed by epiphora caused by punctal occlusion. Similarly, patients with meibomian gland dysfunction, blepharitis, or mucin deficiencies are unlikely to benefit from punctal occlusion unless a concomitant aqueous deficiency exists. Using collagen plugs as a trial/diagnostic initial procedure is preferable.[48,49] The collagen plugs dissolve over a few days, providing adequate time to consider the value of progressing to silicon plugs for semipermanent effects. Silicone plugs will give long-term results if they don't spontaneously extrude. The advantage of collagen plug trials is that adverse symptoms of epiphora will be short term.

A decision to try punctal occlusion should be based on a complete tear deficiency examination with special consideration on Schirmer's, cotton thread, and fluorescein dilution tests for aqueous production.

Positive results are more apparent if both upper and lower puncta are occluded for the most symptomatic eye. Local anesthetic and jeweler's forceps will assist implantation, although simple tweezers can be used successfully without anesthetic.[48,49] It is important to advance the implant well into the canaliculus to reduce the tendency for extrusion. Because itch, irritation, and even abrasion of the ocular surface may occur, careful follow-up is indicated. Successful punctal occlusion can reduce the need for and increase the efficiency of tear supplements.[48,49]

Conclusion

Dry eye conditions are difficult to classify, especially marginal conditions. Currently available methods for dry eye condition examination and classification may yield only a general diagnosis, and management approaches specific to particular dry eye conditions may not be available. This less than satisfactory situation will be alleviated by refinement of clinical tests for dry eye so that diagnostic accuracy and differential diagnosis of dry eye are possible.[50,51]

Contact lens practitioners must deal with the additional complication of interpreting lens and tissue changes occurring in a range of marginal dry eye conditions that are difficult to differentiate. Nevertheless, a comprehensive approach to prefitting examinations will permit appropriate prophylaxis and an equally thorough attitude toward aftercare can be the basis for effective management of dry–eye-related contact lens wear.

References

1. Greiner JV, Allansmith MR: Effect of contact lens wear on the conjunctival mucous system, *Ophthalmol* 88:821-832, 1981.
2. Lemp MA: Surfacing abnormalities, *Int Ophthalmol Clin* 13:191-197, 1973.
3. Holly FJ: The preocular tear film, *Cont IOL Med J* 4:134-142, 1978.
4. Kline LN, DeLuca TJ: Effect of gel lens wear on the precorneal tear film, *Int Cont Lens Clin* 2:56-62, 1975.
5. Cedarstaff TH, Tomlinson A: A comparative study of tear evaporation rates and water content of soft contact lenses, *Am J Optom Physiol Opt* 60:167-174, 1983.
6. Stuchell RN, Farris RL, Mandel ID: Basal and reflex human tear analysis II. Chemical analysis: lactoferrin and lysozyme, *Ophthalmol* 88:858-862, 1981.
7. Andrasko G: Hydrogel dehydration in various environments, *Int Cont Lens Clin* 10:22-28, 1983.
8. Hill RM: The "phantom thickness" factor, *Int Cont Lens Clin* 10:53-55, 1983.
9. Refojo MF, Leong F-L: Water pervaporation through silicone rubber contact lenses: a possible cause of complications, *Cont IOL Med J* 7:226-233, 1981.
10. Tsubai T: Contact lens and the potential dry eye. Part I. Blurs of the HCL surface, *Contacto* 27:22-30, 1983.
11. McMonnies CW, Ho A: Patient history in screening for dry eye conditions, *J Am Optom Assoc* 58:296-301, 1987.

12. Molenaar NJ: Response effects of "formal" characteristics of questions. In Dijkstra W, van der Zouwen J (eds): *Response Behaviour in the Survey Interview,* London, 1982, Academic Press, 66.
13. Henderson JW: Keratoconjunctivitis sicca, *Am J Ophthalmol* 33:197-223, 1950.
14. Stewart C: Functional blinking and contact lenses, *Am J Optom Arch Am Acad Optom* 45:687-691, 1968
15. Korb D: The role of blinking in successful contact lens wear, *Int Cont Lens Clin* 1:59-71, 1974.
16. Collins MJ, Brown B, Bowman KJ: Short term responses to soft contact lens corrections for presbyopia, *Clin Exp Optom* 72:55-60, 1989.
17. McMonnies CW: Contact lens aftercare: A detailed analysis, *Clin Exp Optom* 70:121-127, 1987.
18. Holly FJ, Lemp MA: Tear physiology and dry eyes, *Surv Ophthalmol* 22:69-87, 1977.
19. McCulley JP, Sciallis GF: Meibomian keratoconjunctivitis, *Am J Ophthalmol* 84:788-793, 1977.
20. Mackie IA, Seal DV: The questionably dry eye, *Br J Ophthalmol* 65: 2-9, 1981.
21. Lemp MA, Mahmood MA, Weiler HH: Association of rosacea and keratoconjunctivitis sicca, *Arch Ophthalmol* 102:556-557, 1984.
22. Liu D, Stasior OG: Lower eyelid laxity and ocular symptoms, *Am J Ophthalmol* 95:545-551, 1983.
23. Wright HJ, MacAdam DB: *Clinical thinking and practice: Diagnosis and Decisions in Patient Care,* New York, 1979, Churchill Livingstone, 76-77.
24. McMonnies CW: Key questions in a dry eye history, *J Am Optom Assoc* 57:512-517, 1986.
25. McMonnies CW, Ho A: Responses to a dry eye questionnaire from a normal population, *J Am Optom Assoc* 58:588-591, 1987.
26. McMonnies CW: Allergic complications in contact lens wear, *Int Cont Lens Clinic* 5:182-189, 1978.
27. McCulley JP, Dougherty JM, Deneau DG: Classification of chronic blepharitis, *Ophthalmol* 89:1173-1180, 1982.
28. Lamberts DW, Foster CS, Perry HD: Schirmer test after topical anesthesia and the tear meniscus height in normal eyes, *Arch Ophthalmol* 97:1082-1085, 1979.
29. Josephson JE: Appearance of the preocular tear film lipid layer, *Am J Optom Physiol Opt* 60:883-887, 1983.
30. McMonnies CW, Ho A: Marginal dry eye diagnosis: History versus biomicroscopy. In Holly FJ (ed): *The Preocular Tear Film in Health, Disease and Contact Lens Wear,* Lubbock (Texas), 1986, Dry Eye Institute, 32-40.
31. Mishima S, Gasset A, Klyce D Jr, Baum JL: Determination of tear volume and tear flow, *Inv Ophthalmol* 5:264-276, 1966.
32. Furukawa RE, Polse KA: Changes in tear flow accompanying aging, *Am J Optom Physiol Opt* 55:69-74, 1978.
33. Katz J, Kaufman HE: Corneal exposure during sleep (nocturnal lagophthalmos), *Arch Ophthalmol* 95:449-453 , 1977.
34. Prause JU, Frost-Larsen K, Isager H. Manthorpe R: Tear absorption into the filter-paper strip used in the Schirmer I test, *Acta Ophthalmol* 60:70-78, 1982.
35. Feldman F. Wood MW: Evaluation of the Schirmer tear test, *Can J Ophthalmol* 14:257-259, 1979.
36. van Bijsterveld OP: Diagnostic tests in the sicca syndrome, *Arch Ophthalmol* 82:10-14, 1969.
37. Clinch TE, Benedetto DA, Felberg NT, Laibson PR: Schirmer's test: A closer look, *Arch Ophthalmol* 101:1383-1386, 1983.
38. Jordan A, Baum J: Basic tear flow: Does it exist? *Ophthalmol* 87:920-930, 1980.
39. Lemp MA: Recent developments in dry eye management, *Ophthalmol* 94:1299-1304, 1987.

40. Kurihashi K, Yanagihara N, Honda Y: A modified Schirmer test: The fine-thread method for measuring lacrimation, *J Pediatr Ophthalmol* 14:390-398, 1977.

41. Carey S: Tear film stabilizer, *Contacto* 27:21-23, 1983.

42. Barber JC: Management of the patient with dry eyes, *Cont IOL Med J* 3:10-15, 1977.

43. Lemp MA: Recent developments in dry eye management, *Ophthalmol* 94:1299-1304, 1987.

44. Henriquz AS, Korb DR: Meibomian glands and contact lens wear, *Br J Ophthalmol* 65:108-111, 1981.

45. Korb DR, Korb JE: Fitting to achieve normal blinking and lid action, *Int Cont Lens Clin* 1:57-70, 1974.

46. Korb DR, Korb JE, The American Research Laboratories: *How to Blink Correctly*, Brochure—Sola/Barnes Hind, 1988.

47. McMonnies CW: *Blinking and contact lens performance*, Practice Brochure, 1969.

48. Caffery B: How to approach punctal occlusion, *Cont Lens Spec* 9:49, 1994.

49. Bockin DG: How to perform punctal occlusion, *Cont Lens Spec* 8:30-32, 1993.

50. Albietz JM, Golding TR: Differential diagnosis and management of common dry eye subtypes, *Clin Exp Optom* 77:244-260, 1994.

51. Golding TR, Brennan NA: Diagnostic accuracy and inter-correlation of clinical tests for dry eye, *Inv Ophthalmol Vis Sci (Suppl)* 34:823, 1993.

Appendix 2-1[46]

Did you know that many people with visual problems develop incorrect blinking habits? As a contact lens wearer, correct blinking is especially important to you.

If you blink partially or incorrectly, the area of the cornea not covered by your contact lens can dry. Your eyes may feel itchy, tired, or heavy. You also may develop a burning sensation.

Sometimes the drying makes contact lens wear difficult from the beginning, but usually the effects of dryness don't develop until after months or years of wear. If the dryness becomes severe enough, wearing contact lenses is no longer possible.

Blinking correctly can maximize your ability to wear contact lenses comfortably, for a long time.

Experts in the contact lens industry have developed exercises designed to eliminate improper blinking by substituting a natural, fluid movement that uses your eye muscles correctly.

Steps to Correct Blinking*

Relax

To relax your eyes, you must relax your whole body. Keeping your head straight and erect, place your fingertips at the corner of your eyelids and focus your eyes straight ahead. Don't concentrate on looking ahead when your eyes are closed. That tends to force unnatural eye movement, which can cause muscle tension.

Close

In a gentle, smooth motion, close your lids. If you feel tension through your fingertips, try closing your eyes in "slow motion," as if you're falling off to sleep. As your eyes close, don't let them turn downward; rather, let them drift up as the lid moves downward to close.

Pause

With your eyes closed, pause for a count of three. Feel the sensation of complete closure of your eyes. If you're doing the exercise properly, the muscles will relax and allow the eyes to drift upward as in sleep.

Open

Slowly open your eyes slightly wider than usual. Just slightly, without forcing the muscles or wrinkling your brow.

---

*Reprinted with permission from Sola/Barnes Hind, 1988.

Pause

With your eyes wide open, pause for a count of two.

Repeat

Do the exercise again in this rhythm: close, pause, pause, pause; open, pause, pause; close, pause, pause, pause; open, pause, pause.

Practice

Performing this exercise 15 times a day, with 10 correct blinks each (or as your eye care practitioner prescribes) will help you learn to blink correctly. Three to eight weeks of correct practice should improve your blinking habits significantly.

Note: Some new contact lens wearers experience blurred vision with a full correct blink when excess tears move over the contact lens. There may be a temptation to inhibit blinking or to blink partially. If this happens, tell your eye care practitioner.

The ideal blink

Your goal is a complete, fluid, natural-looking blink. Remember the following tips:
1. Practice this smooth movement at 5-second intervals (that's how frequently most people blink).
2. Learn to blink when you change the direction of your gaze (rather than when you're looking at someone).
3. Hold your head slightly forward with your chin down (it gives a more natural appearance).
4. Practice the blinking exercise faithfully (achieving the ideal blink will be automatic as a result).

Correct blinking helps ensure sharp vision, improved eye health, and successful contact lens wear.

Appendix 2-2[47]

Blinking and Contact Lens Performance

A guide to greater success with contact lenses

Sometimes poor blink habits are the only reason for not achieving complete success with contact lenses.

At all times blinking should assist lens performance. The number of blinks is not as important as the quality or type of blink.

The type of blink required for optimum contact lens performance has the following characteristics:

1. An efficient blink is *complete* or *full*, meaning that the top lid lightly touches the bottom lid.
2. An efficient blink is *relaxed* or *light*, involving only the eyelid muscles. The muscles of the eyebrows or the cheeks are not involved.
3. An efficient blink is *quick* or *reflex*, meaning that minimum delay is involved. The normal full blink should only take one third of a second.
4. Finally, an efficient blink is *confident* and *natural* and looks that way to other people.

A good quality blink helps contact lens performance in a number of ways:

1. A good blink evens out the tear layer on the lens' front surface so that the clearest vision is obtained.
2. A good blink lifts the lens into position in front of the pupil. Often the lens tends to fall down between blinks but . . .
3. The lens' up and down movement is an important design feature and promotes tear circulation.
4. A good blink may be necessary to provide for tear circulation through a lens fenestration (breathing hole).
5. A good blink helps keep the lens' front surface clean.
6. A good blink also helps eliminate excess moisture from the eye.

Half blinks, awkward blinks, hesitant blinks, and slow blinks, are all inefficient and can result in poor performance despite correctly fitted lenses.

The usual way to detect that someone is wearing contact lenses is to notice that blinking is awkward and unnatural. It is true that the most natural-looking blink should be the one that occurs without conscious effort, that is, automatically.

However, it also is true that by making an effort to blink correctly during practice sessions you can develop good automatic blinking habits.

Practice sessions should be only about 30 to 40 seconds. During a practice session you should aim to produce the required blink about 24 times using conscious control to produce all the required characteristics of an efficient blink presented earlier.

You should manufacture the required type of blink by thinking about these desirable qualities as you practice. Memorize the list before you begin. Recall the sequence, one at a time, as you produce each practice blink: *complete, full, relaxed, light, quick, reflex, confident, natural.*

Practicing once or twice a day is better than not at all. However, for good results you should practice at least 20 times a day for a week. That would be only a total of about 10 to 12 minutes per day. Remembering to take time to do these exercises can be a problem. Wearing your wrist watch on your other arm or some other device can help remind you.

Once efficient blinking habits are established it is likely that they will serve you always. The best time to establish good blinking habits is in the early stages of your adaptation, but blinking practice is worthwhile at any time.

3

Soft Lens Extended Wear

Timothy J. Grant
Robert Terry
Brien A. Holden

Key Terms

extended wear	signs	adverse reactions
hydrogel	symptoms	observations
complications	etiology	

High water content (HWC) hydrogel materials were developed and dispensed as continuous-wear contact lenses in Great Britain in the early 1970s.[1] Subsequently, the U.S. Food and Drug Administration (FDA) approved hydrogel lenses for aphakic and cosmetic continuous wear.[2] Extensive marketing of the products as "30-day" lenses resulted in approximately 21% of all hydrogel lens patients using them on an extended-wear basis.[3] The early enthusiasm for continuous hydrogel lens wear was followed by concern as reports of problems associated with the modality began to appear.[3-7] The early papers[4,5,8] reported epithelial microcysts, acute red eye reaction, vascularization, and the first of the serious ulcers. It also was reported that corneal ulceration was far more prevalent among patients using extended-wear lenses than among patients using lenses on a daily-wear basis.[6] Other researchers reached similar conclusions about the prevalence of extended-wear corneal infections and recommended against the use of steroids until the cause was determined.[7] Data from 1989[9,10] confirmed the risk factors for infection reported in earlier studies.[7]

Concern over the greater risk of ulcerative keratitis in users of extended-wear soft contact lenses led the FDA in May 1989 to recommend a maximum of 7 days' wear before overnight removal and disinfection.[11,12]

In view of these findings, practitioners and patients must exercise great care to prevent serious complications. The practitioner must have a thorough understanding of extended wear's ocular effects and of patient management strategies to prevent problems. In this chapter we identify the etiology, signs and symptoms, treatment, observation, and management of the major hydrogel extended-wear problems.

Definitions

The following definitions are used throughout this chapter:
1. *Daily wear.* Contact lenses used only during waking hours. The lenses are removed, cleaned, and disinfected every night before sleep. The lenses may or may not be replaced after a period of wear on the recommendation of the eye care practitioner.
2. *Flexible wear.* Contact lenses that are worn on a daily basis; however, the patient sleeps in them 1 or 2 nights a week. The lenses are replaced as recommended by the practitioner.
3. *Extended wear.* Lenses used continuously for a prescribed period, for example, 7 days and 6 nights or 14 days and 13 nights consecutively. On the final night, the lenses are removed and discarded or cleaned, disinfected, and reinserted the following morning.

Ocular Effects of Hydrogel Extended-Wear Contact Lenses

Corneal Edema
Etiology
Corneal edema with hydrogel lenses is caused by a reduction in available oxygen below the level required to maintain normal corneal thickness. This swelling's etiology is presumed to be lactic acid accumulation. Hypoxic edema can be induced even under normal (no lens) conditions. For example, corneal thickness increases by about 3% to 4%, on average, during 8 hours of sleep.[13] Hydrogels induced 10% to 15% mean overnight corneal edema and the cornea deswelled only 8% after eye opening.[14] Because all current hydrogel lenses induce 10% or greater overnight corneal edema,[15] they will all cause residual corneal edema during the day.

CLINICAL PEARL

All current hydrogel lenses induce 10% or greater overnight corneal edema.

Signs and Symptoms

In severe cases of acute corneal swelling (>20%) loss of corneal transparency usually occurs.[16] Long-term effects of chronic corneal hypoxia include decreased epithelial thickness and adhesion, stromal thinning, and endothelial polymegethism.[17,18] The signs and significance of the corneal edema levels are summarized in Table 3-1.[16]

The most easily recognizable signs of edema are striae and folds caused by the increase in fluid (water) entering the stroma. Striae appear as fine, vertical, grayish-white lines in the posterior stroma.[16] Striae attributable to hydrogel lens wear are usually single lines, whereas rigid gas-permeable (RGP) striae occur in clumps.[19]

The occurrence of folds is a sign that buckling has occurred in Descemet's membrane and the endothelium. Folds appear as black lines when viewed using direct focal illumination with the biomicroscope.[16]

Patients generally report few symptoms unless edema is severe. Slight discomfort and blurred vision on waking may be reported, though these symptoms are usually transient. With chronic high levels of daytime edema (>8%) patients will eventually experience decreased vision, glare, photophobia, and colored halos around lights; vascularization will occur.[20]

Observation

Biomicroscopic observation of striae and folds is best conducted using a parallelepiped at medium magnification (16× to 20×) with white light. Striae can be observed in the central and peripheral stroma, although they are more easily noted in the central position using the pupil as a background.

TABLE 3-1
Corneal Edema Levels

Corneal Swelling	Signs	Significance
<2%	Undetectable	Unknown
2% to 5%	Some initial striae	Chronic changes
>5%	Vertical striae	Chronic hypoxic effects
>8%	Posterior folds, striae	Acute edema
>20%	Loss of transparency, folds, striae	Pathological

Management

After the first night of hydrogel extended wear, patients should be seen within 3 hours of waking. If folds are observed after 1 hour of open-eye lens wear, extended wear should be discontinued with that lens. If striae are observed, the patient should be monitored more closely. Persistent daytime striae and folds are unacceptable and necessitate discontinuation of the current mode of extended wear.

CLINICAL PEARL

After the first night of hydrogel extended wear, patients should be seen within 3 hours of waking.

A number of alternative strategies exist for alleviating daytime edema caused by extended wear. The lens' Dk/L should be increased by using a higher water content lens or a thinner hydrogel lens. Alternatively, the number of nights of wear can be reduced, or the patient can be refitted with a high Dk/L RGP lens[20] (see Figures 3-1 and 3-2).

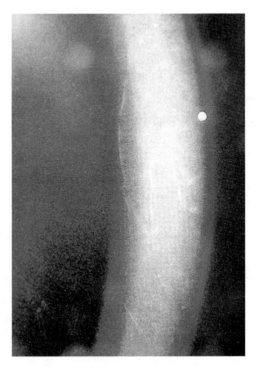

FIGURE 3-1 Corneal striae on eye opening after overnight lens wear.

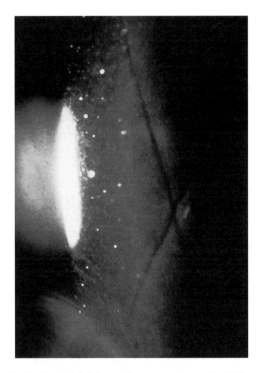

FIGURE 3-2   Endothelial folds with approximately 15% corneal edema.

Epithelial Microcysts

Etiology

Microcysts are among the best clinical indicators of chronic induced hypoxia.[21] It is thought that microcysts are dead or aging cells trapped in the epithelium and brought to the corneal surface at a slower rate than normal epithelial cells.[22]

CLINICAL PEARL

Microcysts are among the best clinical indicators of chronic induced hypoxia.

Although microcysts can occur with daily wear of hydrogel lenses[23] they are almost always observed in patients wearing soft lenses on any regimen that involves overnight wear. In general, as the number of nights that lenses are worn while sleeping increases, so do the number of microcysts. It has not yet been established whether microcysts result solely from hypoxia or whether the acid shift resulting from CO_2 accumulation contributes.[21]

Signs and Symptoms

Microcysts are small (15µm to 50µm), irregular, refractile dots observed in the epithelium and usually seen in the cornea's central and paracentral regions.[24] Although the number of microcysts varies, the average number encountered with extended wear of current hydrogel lenses is 30 to 40.[23]

In most cases patients are asymptomatic. Very occasionally, microcysts will cause a small amount of epithelial staining and discomfort. If the number is large (>200) and the epithelium is disrupted, vision also may be slightly compromised.

Observation

The best method of observing microcysts with the biomicroscope is to use marginal direct retroillumination with 30× to 40× magnification. Microcysts display reversed illumination when observed in this manner (i.e., when observed against a background, the microcyst's dark side appears on the opposite side to the background).[24]

To assist in distinguishing between tear debris and microcysts the patient should be instructed to blink frequently.

Management

Management of microcysts varies according to their number. It has been suggested that if fewer than 50 are observed, no action is necessary; however, the patient should be closely monitored.[24] In our experience, although as many as 80 microcysts can occur without epithelial staining, it is highly desirable to reduce the number of microcysts to below 10.[25]

Progressive strategies to avoid microcysts include:
1. Using higher Dk/L lenses (over 50×10^{-9})
2. Reducing the number of nights of wear or returning the patient to daily wear
3. Refitting the patient with high Dk RGP lenses

When patients discontinue lens wear, the number of microcysts initially increases, reaching a maximum 1 to 2 weeks after discontinuation. Full epithelial recovery usually takes 6 to 8 weeks following cessation of lens wear.[17,24]

Epithelial Vacuoles

Etiology

Vacuoles are generally larger and more discrete than microcysts, varying in size from 20 µm to 50 µm.[24] They are round with distinct edges and display unreversed illumination.[24] They can occur in discrete spots or in groups and are found with all modes of lens wear, although they generally become more numerous as the number of nights of wear increases. Vacuoles also can be found in nonwearing patients.

Signs and Symptoms

Patients are asymptomatic and vacuoles do not cause any compromise to vision or lens comfort. Vacuoles occur within the same time frame as microcysts, but are not cyclical and do not temporarily increase in number when lens wear has ceased. An incidence of 32% among continuous-wear patients has been reported.[24] We have found that all patients have vacuoles within 1 year of commencement of hydrogel extended wear.

Observation

The method of observation is the same as that for microcysts; however, vacuoles show an unreversed illumination effect (i.e., the vacuole's dark side is on the same side as the dark background)[24] (Figures 3-3 and 3-4).

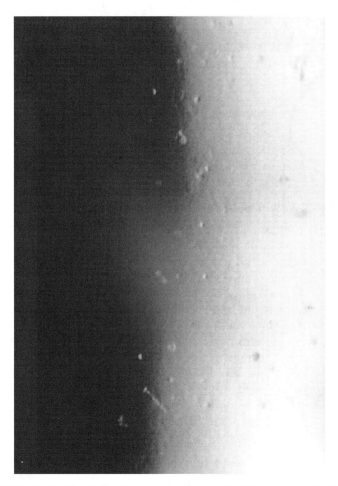

FIGURE 3-3 Epithelial microcysts observed with marginal retroillumination, demonstrating the reversed illumination effect.

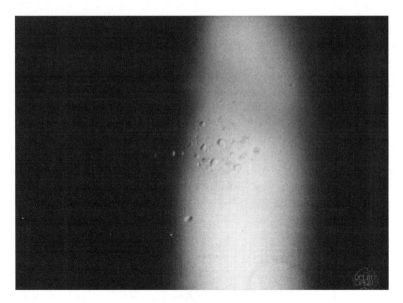

FIGURE 3-4 Epithelial vacuoles observed with direct retroillumination.

Management

Vacuoles should be noted and monitored. Discontinuation of lens wear is usually unnecessary if vacuoles are few in number. However, if the vacuoles coalesce and cause epithelial staining, lens wear should be discontinued until resolution.

Endothelial Polymegethism

Etiology

The normal endothelium is a regular, uniform mosaic in which both cell size and shape are consistent. Polymegethism is a term used to describe the variation in endothelial cell size. The coefficient of variation (i.e., standard deviation of cell area divided by the mean cell area) is one measure of polymegethism. Endothelial variation normally increases with age; however, a greater degree of polymegethism and a more rapid rate of change have been reported in association with both daily and extended wear of hydrogel lenses and with long-term daily PMMA wear.[21,26-30]

Polymegethism's etiology is unclear. One hypothesis proposes that changes in cell morphology are caused by a reduction in stromal pH during lens wear associated with hypoxia-related lactic acid accumulation or a reduction in CO_2 efflux.[31,32]

Signs and Symptoms

Although polymegethism commences soon after lens wear begins, it is initially asymptomatic. The occurrence of corneal exhaustion syndrome (CES) has been reported, in which long-term lens wearers with high degrees of polymegethism experience decreased lens tolerance and a significantly lower rate of corneal deswelling.[33,34]

Observation

The endothelium is observed with specular reflection at 30× to 40× magnification. The angle between the observation and illumination arms should vary between 40 and 65 degrees depending on the area of the endothelium being viewed. Maximum illumination and magnification and good slit lamp optical quality are necessary. Observation and grading of endothelial polymegethism should be carried out at every patient visit.

Management

It was found[35] that in a group of long-term hydrogel extended-wear patients discontinuation of lens wear for 6 months resulted in a slight but statistically insignificant reduction in polymegethism.

Polymegethism is a difficult management issue. If a patient has a great degree of polymegethism, caution should be exercised in allowing extended wear. Recording changes in polymegethism can only become consistent with repetition, and are best made "masked" to the previous results.

Endothelial Blebs

Etiology

Blebs are black, nonreflecting areas that appear in the endothelial mosaic within minutes of a hydrogel lens being placed on the eye.[36]

The probable cause of the bleb response is a local acidic pH change near the endothelium.[37] Blebs are thought to result from local edema that causes the posterior of the endothelial cell to bulge toward the aqueous.[38,39]

Signs and Symptoms

Blebs are asymptomatic, and no clinical significance has been attached to them. The bleb response peaks 20 to 30 minutes after the lens is placed on the eye, and after approximately 60 minutes of wear the response subsides to a very low level. Blebs disappear within minutes of lens removal.[39] With extended wear, the response diminishes to an almost imperceptible level after 4 or 5 days.[39]

Observation

The bleb response is most easily seen in the endothelial midperiphery using direct illumination with a setting of approximately 60 degrees between the illumination and the observation tube. Specular reflection and the maximum possible slit lamp magnification and illumination should be used.

Corneal Exhaustion Syndrome (CES)
Etiology

In 1988 researchers described a condition in which long-term wearers of low oxygen transmissibility lenses (PMMA and thick (0.15 mm) HEMA) developed intolerance to their lenses.[40] CES patients subjected to a contact–lens-induced hypoxic stress test manifested abnormally high corneal swelling and slower deswelling.

It was proposed that the long-term chronic hypoxia associated with PMMA and thick HEMA lens wear resulted in endothelial cell layer dysfunction and a concomitant reduction in the endothelium's capacity to regulate corneal swelling. Although the syndrome has not yet been documented with hydrogel extended wear, we believe it will become increasingly prevalent among long-term hydrogel extended-wear patients.

Signs and Symptoms

The CES patients manifested significant changes in posterior corneal appearance, including an irregular and distorted endothelial cell mosaic, a reduction in individual cellular clarity, high degrees of polymegethism, and faint posterior stromal opacification.[40] These CES patients reported decreased comfort, edema after 6 to 8 hours of wear, and reduced lens tolerance.

Observation

The biomicroscopic examination techniques of direct focal illumination and specular reflection should be used to assess the integrity of the deep stroma and the endothelial cell layer. The detection of obvious changes in the endothelial cell mosaic should alert the practitioner to the possibility of CES.

Management

At signs of changes to the endothelial mosaic, appropriate steps should be undertaken to prevent the onset of CES. If the patient is to continue with extended wear, it is recommended that high Dk (i.e., 100×10^{-11} (cm^2 × ml 0$_2$) / (sec × ml × mm Hg)) rigid gas-permeable lenses be prescribed.[40]

Epithelial Damage (Corneal Staining)
Etiology

The intact corneal epithelium is a barrier against trauma, pathogens, and chemicals. Any insult to the epithelium may damage cells or increase cellular permeability. Dyes such as sodium fluorescein demonstrate increased cellular permeability; rose bengal, on the other hand, stains dead and damaged cells.

The patterns of staining encountered with hydrogel extended wear vary markedly and the depth can range from a single cell to full epithelial thickness. The principal types of staining are presented in Table 3-3.

Signs and Symptoms

The patient presenting with epithelial trauma may be asymptomatic or may experience discomfort ranging from a slight awareness and a burning, gritty sensation to severe pain and lens intolerance.

Observation

Epithelial staining is best assessed following the instillation of sodium fluorescein with a yellow filter (Wratten Filter #12) placed over the objective of the slit lamp biomicroscope and cobalt blue light (Wratten Filter #47B) placed over the illumination system. All patients who present for aftercare visits should have their lenses removed to allow biomicroscopic examination of corneal integrity using sodium fluorescein. Many cases of epithelial cell damage cannot easily be seen, nor can the depth and extent of the epithelial cell damage be assessed accurately with white light. The grading scales[25] for staining used at the Cornea & Contact Lens Research Unit (CCLRU), School of Optometry, University of New South Wales, Australia, are presented in Table 3-2.

Management

Management of corneal staining depends on its type, depth, and extent. The following guidelines have been suggested for the duration of lens removal required for various depths of corneal staining[41]:

1. 24 hours if slight stromal diffusion of fluorescein occurs over a limited area (Depth Grade 2)
2. 2 to 3 days if moderate stromal diffusion of fluorescein is observed (Depth Grade 3)
3. At least 7 days if immediate and widespread stromal diffusion of fluorescein occurs (Depth Grade 4)

A cornea with moderate to severe staining should be reexamined after 2 days to confirm that the epithelium has healed before lens wear resumes. If lenses are worn during the recovery stage, the time required for healing will be longer and the chance of a corneal infection will increase. The cornea should be examined again 2 or 3 days after lens wear has recommenced (see Figures 3-5 through 3-7).

TABLE 3-2

CCLRU Grading for Epithelial Staining

Grade	Extent	Grade	Depth
0	Absent	0	Absent
1	1% to 15% surface involvement	1	Superficial epithelial involvement
2	16% to 30% surface involvement	2	Stromal glow present within 30 seconds
3	31% to 45% surface involvement	3	Immediate localized stromal glow
4	46% or greater surface involvement	4	Immediate diffuse stromal glow

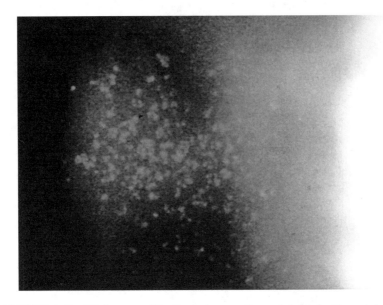

FIGURE 3-5 High magnification observation of dehydration staining.

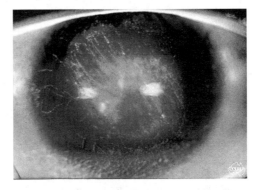

FIGURE 3-6 Widespread toxic staining pattern.

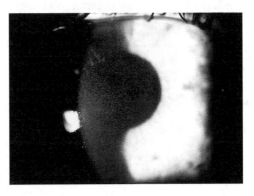

FIGURE 3-7 Severe foreign body staining pattern.

TABLE 3-3

Treatment Alternatives for Epithelial Staining

Cause	Corneal Location	Description	Treatment Alternatives
Dehydration	Central, superior, inferior	White flakelike superficial punctate to full-thickness epithelial erosions	• Increase lens thickness • Decrease water content • Change to RGP lenses • Cease lens wear
Toxic	Usually total surface involvement	Superficial punctate staining	• Change care regimen • Disposable lenses (no care regimen) • Change lens material
Exposure	Inferior arcuate band	Coalescent and punctate staining involving the cornea and conjunctiva	• Optimize lens design • Blink instructions • In-eye lubricant • Change to RGP lenses • Cease lens wear
Mechanical	Localized depending upon cause (e.g., foreign body, damaged lens)	Varies in depth and extent	• Optimize lens design • Replace damaged lens • Remove foreign body
Hypoxia	Variable	Varies from superficial punctate to confluent patches	• Reduce lens thickness • Increase water content • Flatten base curve • Decrease wear time • Change to RGP lenses • Cease lens wear

Treatment alternatives for epithelial staining have been summarized in Table 3-3.[42]

Endothelial Bedewing

Etiology

Bedewing is described as a cluster of droplets (perhaps leukocytes) on the posterior endothelial surface. The clusters generally consist of 20 to 50 droplets and are observed on the inferior endothelium approximately one third of the distance below the pupil margin at the 6 o'clock position.[43]

Their significance is not yet fully understood, although it is suggested that bedewing is a low-grade inflammatory response consisting of inflammatory cells resting on the endothelium.[43]

Signs and Symptoms

Bedewing is most often seen following an inflammatory incident such as acute red eye.[43] The condition may be asymptomatic or accompanied by discomfort, photophobia, and decreased vision.[43]

Observation

Bedewing is best observed using marginal retroillumination under medium magnification with a moderately wide parallelepiped. Observation is more difficult in patients with dark irides.

Management

Bedewing is a benign condition that may indicate a previous inflammatory episode. Patients do not need to reduce wearing time if asymptomatic bedewing is observed; however, it can take 3 to 6 months to resolve. If symptoms are present, however, wearing time should be reduced; it may be necessary to return the patient to daily wear.

Corneal Infiltrates

Etiology

Infiltrates are an inflammatory response in which cells released from the limbal vasculature invade the cornea.[44] Contact–lens-induced infiltrates may be lymphocytes; they also may be phagocytic macrophages or other invading inflammatory tissue cells. They are found in a variety of conditions including acute red eye, corneal ulceration, infections (e.g., keratoconjunctivitis), localized trauma, solution sensitivity, and prolonged hypoxia. They also may occur because of mechanical pressure from a tight lens. The stimulus may therefore be mechanical, toxic, microbiological, or chemical.[44]

Signs and Symptoms

Infiltrates can be epithelial, subepithelial, or stromal.[44-46] They typically appear as whitish-gray spots and patches. In asymptomatic patients they are commonly located in the superior cornea, covered by the upper lid.[46,47] They may either be diffuse (ill-defined borders) or focal (localized with well-defined borders).

Signs and symptoms of infiltrates include ocular irritation, lens discomfort, foreign body sensation, photophobia, lacrimation, and localized conjunctival and limbal vessel hyperemia. Infiltrates also may be asymptomatic.

Observation

Infiltrates can involve all regions of the cornea. They can easily be overlooked, particularly if the patient is asymptomatic or has vague symptoms. A thorough and systematic approach to corneal observation is the best safeguard against overlooking such conditions.

Contact–lens-induced infiltrates generally are located within 2 mm to 3 mm of the limbus. Focal infiltrates usually are seen close to the limbus and in the conjunctiva immediately adjacent to the limbus. A close examination of the limbus at all aftercare visits is essential, because infiltrates are sometimes difficult to observe in this region.

Focal infiltrates are revealed under white light and medium magnification. Diffuse infiltrates are even more difficult to observe, requiring a parallelepiped with medium magnification and bright illumination. The affected corneal areas appear whitish and hazy, and when viewed with indirect retroillumination will have an "orange peel" appearance.

When observing infiltrates, care should be taken not to confuse them with early changes associated with arcus senilis. Detailed baseline examination will help resolve any confusion.

Management

The presence of infiltrates necessitates discontinuation of lens wear and monitoring of the patient until the infiltrates have fully resolved. Lens wear should not be resumed while infiltrates are present. If a loss of epithelial integrity occurs over an area of infiltration, infectious keratitis should be assumed and appropriate treatment commenced without delay. Wherever possible, the cause of the infiltrates must be determined, because treatment varies according to etiology. Symptoms usually resolve before the infiltrates completely disappear. As infiltrates resolve, they change color to a whitish-brown and become granular in appearance. When this occurs, the infiltrates will fully resolve within 2 weeks. New lenses should be issued and lens wear restricted to a daily basis for at least 2 weeks before recommencement of extended wear. If infiltrates recur with hydrogel lens wear, refitting with rigid gas-permeable lenses should be considered (see Figure 3-8).

Contact Lens Acute Red Eye (CLARE)
Etiology

The contact lens acute red eye (CLARE) reaction in hydrogel extended wear is a common and disturbing inflammatory response. The annual incidence in our extended-wear studies is between 4% and 30% and depends on lens type, care regimen, and lens replacement frequency.[48]

Although CLARE's etiology is not well defined, some suggested contributing factors include:

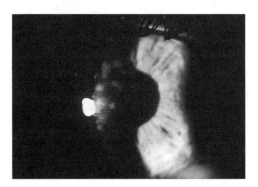

FIGURE 3-8 Focal and diffuse central stromal infiltrates.

1. A toxic response to cellular debris trapped beneath an immobile lens[49]
2. Trauma caused by a lens that fits poorly or does not move adequately[2]
3. Bacterial contamination[50]
4. An allergic/toxic response to long-term exposure to care systems and their preservatives[51]
5. Residues left on the lens after manufacture (unpublished data)
6. Protein accumulation in or on the lens[52]
7. Physical stress (e.g., a cold, influenza, or general debilitation) (unpublished data)
8. Acute hypoxia[50]

CCLRU studies have shown that CLARE can occur at any time during extended wear, although the response is most commonly observed within the first 3 months of wear. Some patients experience recurring episodes that may necessitate discontinuation of lens wear.

Signs and Symptoms

Contact lens acute red eye is typically unilateral and occurs around 2 AM to 4 AM. The patient wakes with ocular pain, extreme photophobia, lacrimation, and intense conjunctival and limbal hyperemia.[45]

Signs include subepithelial infiltrates that may be diffuse or focal. The infiltrates usually are found within 2 mm or 3 mm of the limbus, although in severe cases there may be widespread corneal involvement. Other indicators of contact lens acute red eye are bulbar conjunctival hyperemia (usually involving the whole eye) and limbal injection. Less severe cases may exhibit only localized injection of the conjunctiva and limbus. In these cases infiltrates are observed only in the corneal region immediately adjacent to the conjunctival and limbal injection. Sodium fluorescein pooling is occasionally observed if the CLARE has been associated with debris trapped between the lens and cornea, but obvious epithelial staining is rare. A summary of CLARE's signs and symptoms is given in Table 3-4.

TABLE 3-4
Contact Lens Acute Red Eye (CLARE)

Signs	Symptoms
Unilateral	Awakened at 3 to 5 AM
Infiltrates (focal or diffuse)	Pain
Conjunctival hyperemia	Photophobia
Limbal injection	Lacrimation

Observation

The effects of contact lens acute red eye can be observed under room illumination. Conjunctival hyperemia, photophobia, and discomfort will be noted.

Because slit lamp illumination may cause the patient discomfort, a drop of anesthetic may be instilled to relieve symptoms and allow a thorough corneal examination. Moderate magnification should be used with a parallelepiped using white light. The use of sodium fluorescein, cobalt-blue light, and the Wratten #12 filter is essential to determine if epithelial staining over areas of infiltration has occurred. Care should be taken to ensure that the anesthetic and sodium fluorescein are sterile before instillation.

Management

Although contact lens acute red eye is not a sight-threatening condition, it is painful and seems to recur. The patient should be made aware of the possibility of experiencing acute red eye and instructed to remove the lens immediately and consult his or her practitioner as soon as possible if acute red eye occurs. Repeated occurrences usually necessitate discontinuation of lens wear.

CLARE does not warrant therapeutic intervention. As mentioned previously, however, it is important to distinguish CLARE from infection. Any epithelial defect with underlying infiltrates must be assumed infectious and appropriate therapy commenced immediately.

All infiltrates should fully resolve before lens wear resumes. Usually this takes 2 or 3 weeks, although in some cases it may take as long as 3 months. New lenses should be fitted at the resumption of lens wear. They should be worn on a daily-wear basis for a minimum of 2 weeks while the patient's progress is monitored. A return to extended wear may then be possible.

Regular replacement of lenses decreases CLARE's incidence but does not completely prevent the condition. CCLRU studies report a 5% to 30% yearly incidence of acute red eye with nonreplaced hydrogel extended-wear lenses of varying water contents.[48] The incidence can be reduced to 4% if lenses are regularly replaced (every 1 or 2 weeks). Adequate lens movement, correct lens care and maintenance, and a reduction in nights sleeping in the lenses also assist in the prevention of contact lens acute red eye[48] (see Figure 3-9).

Ulcerative Keratitis

Etiology

Ulcerative keratitis, the most serious and sight-threatening condition associated with hydrogel extended wear, was first reported in the 1970s.[4,5,8,52] The incidence of serious corneal infection is estimated to

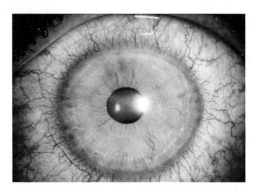

FIGURE 3-9 Contact lens acute red eye.

be 1 in 3000 and to have a five-fold greater risk with extended wear than with daily wear.[7]

An annual incidence between 0.03% and 0.21% of ulcerative keratitis with hydrogel extended wear has been reported.[10,54] Furthermore, it is estimated that hydrogel extended-wear patients are at 10 to 15 times greater risk of developing ulcerative keratitis than daily lens wearers.[9] A greater risk also has been reported with overnight use of daily-wear lenses and with patients who smoke or attend to care and maintenance infrequently. An incidence of approximately 3% sterile peripheral ulcers occurs with hydrogel extended lens wearers, regardless of lens type or replacement schedule.[55] The etiology of these contact–lens-related sterile peripheral ulcers is unclear, but they are similar to *Staphylococcus* toxin ulcers.[56]

A compromised epithelium resulting from hypoxia is a significant contributor to this condition.[21] Reduced epithelial adhesion may be involved.[18] Other factors associated with ulcers include lens handling,[57,58] inappropriate antibiotics,[58] associated eye diseases such as keratoconjunctivitis and blepharitis,[59] diabetes,[60] lens wear in warm climates,[61] delay in lens removal,[62] and inappropriate corticosteroid therapy.[7,57,62]

It is important to distinguish between sterile peripheral ulcers and precursors of serious bacterial corneal infections.[53] The primary diagnosis will be made by examining the appearance, time course, and presence of microorganisms. However, any corneal infiltrate with an overlying epithelial defect must be treated as a potentially serious corneal infection and diagnostic measures and therapy commenced immediately.

Signs and Symptoms

The most obvious sign is acute inflammation. The patient will exhibit an extremely hyperemic conjunctiva, associated with pain and photophobia. Mucopurulent discharge is usually absent in sterile ulcers.

In ulcerative keratitis, an epithelial break occurs in conjunction with localized stromal loss. Underlying infiltrates are present, and localized epithelial and stromal edema usually surrounds the ulcerated area. Vision will remain undisturbed unless the ulceration is central or paracentral. In severe cases hypopyon and cells in the anterior chamber may be present.[63]

Symptoms vary from gradual onset of foreign body sensation to extreme pain and distress. In some cases patients may still be able to wear their lenses and experience only mild irritation. Unilateral photophobia is common, although its severity varies considerably.

Observation

Ulceration is best observed using the slit lamp with a diffusing filter, white light, and low magnification. Prudent observation may reveal one or more white spots, often toward the corneal periphery. With magnification and the use of an optic section, the full epithelial thickness loss with stromal involvement can be viewed. Stromal infiltrates will be noted below the epithelial break and the affected area will have a "ground glass" appearance.

On instillation of sodium fluorescein, the epithelial area will stain rapidly, as will the stroma underlying the epithelial break. Sodium fluorescein may cause patients to experience a slight stinging sensation; rose bengal should not be instilled because it will cause discomfort.

Management

The condition must be distinguished from CLARE, which also produces symptoms of conjunctival hyperemia and patient discomfort. Ulcerative keratitis is identified by the presence of an epithelial lesion with stromal involvement and underlying infiltrates. If possible, the patient should have a culture of the affected area taken before drug therapy begins.[63,64]

Initial treatment consists of a broad-spectrum antibiotic while the organism is being identified, followed by drug therapy specific to the organism.[64] Corticosteroids should not be administered.[63,64] When examining the patient, it is important that any object or solution that comes into contact with the affected eye be sterile; any contamination significantly increases the risk to the patient, because the ulcers themselves are usually sterile.

The patient should be referred immediately to a corneal specialist if the practitioner has any doubts about how best to treat the condition.[63]

Above all, practitioners should aim to prevent ulcerative keratitis. This can best be achieved by reducing the number of nights of wear or avoiding sleeping in lenses altogether, increasing the amount of oxygen available to the cornea, and ensuring compliance with adequate care and maintenance systems (Figure 3-10).

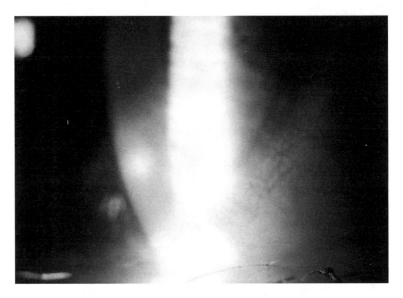

FIGURE 3-10   Culture negative peripheral ulcer.

Giant Papillary Conjunctivitis/Contact–Lens-Related Papillary Conjunctivitis

Etiology

Giant papillary conjunctivitis (GPC)[65,66] and its precursor, contact–lens-related papillary conjunctivitis (CLPC),[67] are the most common causes of permanent discontinuation of soft lens extended wear.[68] These conditions are major problems for wearers and practitioners and often continue to afflict even patients who follow preventive strategies. For example, it was reported[68] that after 2 or more years of hydrogel lens extended wear, 46% of patients wearing HEMA lenses developed GPC. In studies conducted at the CCLRU using a low water content HEMA lens without replacement, similar results were obtained.

CLPC and GPC can be distinguished primarily by the size of the papillae and the severity of symptoms.[66,67] Contact–lens-related papillary conjunctivitis does not develop to the third and fourth stages described previously.[66] Furthermore, if CLPC is closely monitored, the patient can return to lens wear and in some instances, overnight wear.

Possible factors associated with CLPC include lens deposits, duration of lens wear, the lens' age, and the mechanical effects of continual rubbing of the lid by surface deposits.[69-71] Preservatives used in soft contact lens care regimens also may contribute.[69-71]

Hydrogel lenses of different water contents have similar types and amounts of protein on their surfaces, but the majority of the protein is within the matrix of the lens material.[52] Furthermore, the incidence of

CLPC does not correlate with the amount of protein.[72] In view of this evidence, the state of the protein rather than the quantity on the lens may contribute to CLPC's onset. That CLPC and GPC still occur with disposable lenses suggests that a mechanical factor also may contribute to the condition's onset, although daily lens replacement has not yet been tested.

Signs and Symptoms

The classic signs of GPC are giant papillae (>1 mm), flattening and staining of the papillae, mucous strands, severe hyperemia, and occasional corneal involvement (epithelial staining). The signs and symptoms of CLPC are less pronounced, with smaller papillae and less mucous discharge and itching. Lens movement and variable vision also are noted.[66,67]

In the early stages of CLPC the papillae will develop in the lower third of the everted lid area.[66] As the condition progresses, the papillae increase in size and number and total lid involvement occurs.

A comparison of signs and symptoms of GPC and CLPC is presented in Table 3-5.

Observation

Lid eversion should be undertaken at all aftercare visits, preferably at the conclusion of the slit lamp examination because it may cause some patients mild discomfort and induce lacrimation. The slit lamp biomicroscope with diffuse white light should be used to assess hyperemia and mucous response. Instillation of sodium fluorescein and use of blue light facilitate assessment of the papillae's size and number.

TABLE 3-5

Comparative Signs and Symptoms of GPC and CLPC

CLPC	GPC
Signs	
Enlarged papillae	Giant papillae >1 mm (total lid involvement)
Nonuniform appearance	Flattening and staining of papillae
	Mucous strands
Variable hyperemia	Severe hyperemia
	Occasional corneal involvement (staining)
Symptoms	
Intermittent mucus	Excessive mucus
Occasional itchiness	Mild to severe itchiness
Decreased lens tolerance	Lens intolerance
Occasional excessive lens movement	Excessive lens movement
Intermittent variable vision	Variable vision

Management

The recommended course of action for CLPC is to cease lens wear immediately and monitor the patient until the hyperemia, papillae, and mucous response resolve. Symptoms may take as long as 2 months to resolve, and lens wear should not resume until the patient is free of them. Daily lens disposal will alleviate symptoms even while the signs persist. Because daily disposal is expensive, a program of weekly disposal (daily wear) can be attempted after a week of daily disposal.[73] Trials have demonstrated that, although disposable lenses decrease CLPC's incidence, they do not completely prevent it.[48,73]

Recovery from CLPC is slow, and months or even years may elapse before the eyelids return to normal. In some cases the eyelids never completely recover.

In summary, the recommended management strategy for trying to keep CLPC and GPC patients in hydrogel lenses is as follows:
1. Cessation of lens wear for 1 or 2 months or until symptoms resolve
2. Resumption of hydrogel lens wear using disposable lenses on a daily-wear, daily-disposal basis for a week, followed by daily wear, weekly disposal

For both CLPC and GPC, return to extended wear should be discouraged because it will exacerbate the condition. If a patient insists on extended wear, one alternative is to refit him or her with RGP lenses.[74]

Other suggested therapies include the use of Opticrom,[75] vitamin A drops,[76] or topical steroids[63] (Figure 3-11).

Corneal Vascularization

Etiology

Corneal vascularization was a common problem when thick low water content lenses (e.g., 0.2 mm central thickness) were in widespread use. Since the advent of hydrogel lenses with higher oxygen transmissibility it is less frequently encountered. Nevertheless, the appearance of blood vessels within normally avascular corneal tissue is a cause for concern.

Vascularization's etiology is multifactoral. Trauma, peripheral corneal edema, solution sensitivity, vasostimulatory influences from inflammatory cells, and poorly fitting or damaged lenses can all have an influence.[77-79] Lactic acid accumulation in the stroma caused by hypoxia also may be an important factor.[78] A tightly fitting lens may indent the conjunctiva and restrict venous drainage, exacerbating vascularization.[79]

Signs and Symptoms

Vascularization is usually asymptomatic unless vessel growth into the cornea is so extensive that vision is disturbed. It is, however, unusual for vascularization associated with contact lens wear to advance to this stage. In most cases of contact–lens-induced vascularization

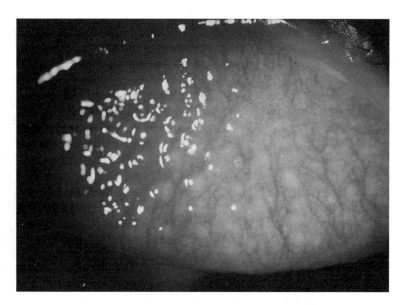

FIGURE 3-11 Giant papillary conjunctivitis.

vessels will be noted approximately 1.5 mm to 2 mm beyond the translucent limbus zone. The vessels can be found in the epithelium or in the stroma. They appear as spikes, branches, or loops of vessels and may occur at any point on the corneal circumference.[80]

Observation

Careful examination of the circumference of the corneo-limbal junction is required to distinguish between limbal and corneal vessels. This is achieved by locating the translucent limbal transition zone using a moderately wide parallelepiped and marginal retroillumination with the slit lamp.[81] Vessels extending beyond the limbal transition zone should be viewed with concern. An eyepiece equipped with a graticule should be used to record the vessel's length for comparison with future observations.

Management

With cessation of lens wear corneal vessels may empty, become ghost vessels, and remain indefinitely. The vessels may regress completely depending upon the stage at which the stimulus to vascularization was removed.[78] The ghost vessels will, however, fill rapidly if the stimulus to vascularization returns.[80]

Continued use of extended-wear hydrogel lenses following vascularization is not recommended unless causes such as hypoxia, solution sensitivity, and trauma have been identified and eliminated. If lens wear resumes, the patient will require careful monitoring to ensure that the condition does not recur[80] (Figure 3-12).

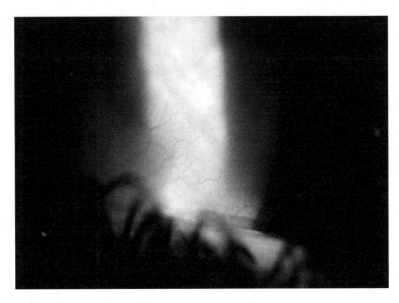

FIGURE 3-12 Corneal vascularization showing vessel extension into the stroma.

Solution Sensitivity

Etiology

Reactions to contact lens care solutions are always possible. The severity of reactions may vary considerably, and diagnosis of the cause is made difficult by the variety of factors that may be involved.

The most common cause of solution sensitivity reaction is the continuous exposure of the eye to preservatives absorbed by the lens material. Lenses absorb preservatives to varying degrees, and those that absorb greater amounts of preservative are most likely to cause a reaction.[82,83]

Acute toxic responses also occur, usually within minutes of lens insertion, and are accompanied by stinging, discomfort, lacrimation, and decreased vision. These symptoms are alleviated by removal of the lenses.

Environmental contaminants such as toxic fumes or heavily polluted air are possible causes of sensitivity reactions. Patients who have a history of allergies are more likely to suffer allergic reactions to preserved solutions, particularly those that have thimerosal[83] or chlorhexidine as ingredients.[84]

Signs and Symptoms

Solution reactions are usually slow to manifest. Characteristic symptoms include an increase in lens-related discomfort, decreased wearing time, and conjunctival hyperemia. If corneal involvement occurs, diffuse punctate staining and infiltrates may be observed and the eyelid also may be affected by increased hyperemia, chemosis, and itchiness.[84,85] Hyperemia and corneal staining are the signs most readily identified by practitioners. Staining will usually resolve at a slower rate than that caused by physical trauma.

Management

The reaction's cause must be determined and then eliminated. The lens should be purged of the solution by soaking it for 24 hours in unpreserved saline that is changed every 6 to 12 hours. Some practitioners may find it more convenient to dispense disposable lenses rather than purge the existing lenses. Solution sensitivity reactions can be avoided with preservative-free regimens. It also is reported that low-toxicity preservatives cause fewer sensitivity problems, although the long-term microbial efficacy of such solutions has not yet been determined.

Bulbar Conjunctival Trauma

Etiology

When there is no pain, conjunctival hyperemia is usually the main indicator to patients that they need to consult their practitioners. A conjunctival reaction may result from mechanical insult caused by the lens or prolonged exposure to lens-related toxic substances or deposits.[86] The most common insult to the conjunctiva caused by a soft lens is either mild abrasion or excessive pressure.

Trauma to the soft lens patient's conjunctiva also may be associated with a tightly fitting or badly shaped lens edge. In such cases the lens can restrict blood flow, indent, or even abrade the conjunctiva. Hyperemia, staining, and occasionally a subconjunctival hemorrhage can occur.[84,85]

Signs and Symptoms

The most obvious sign of conjunctival trauma is hyperemia, ranging from mild injection to severe vessel engorgement, conjunctival chemosis, and a watery discharge. The conjunctival hyperemia associated with a CLARE reaction and infected ulcer are the most severe signs that contact lens practitioners will encounter. Hyperemia and injection caused by other forms of trauma such as foreign bodies also should be considered when examining the contact lens patient.

Symptoms related to primary conjunctival traumas such as those caused by lens edges include vague discomfort with a mild foreign body sensation.

Hyperemia is often confined to the area affected by the lens. The epithelium will stain with sodium fluorescein; rose bengal, if instilled, also may show staining. Sometimes the conjunctiva will be slightly chemotic and an area of sodium fluorescein pooling will be noted that is not typical staining.

When diagnosing contact–lens-associated conjunctival problems, the practitioner must be aware of the possibility of bacterial or viral conjunctivitis. These infections are more likely to occur with patients who do not comply with their care and maintenance regimens. Signs of such infections include purulent mucous or watery discharge, crusty exudate on lid margins, hyperemia, chemosis, and lid edema.[88]

Observation

A thorough conjunctival examination is required with white and blue light and sodium fluorescein. With white light the conjunctiva can be examined for foreign bodies, lacerations, and subconjunctival hemorrhages. An assessment for hyperemia is best conducted with white light.

Sodium fluorescein is essential for the examination of the conjunctiva. Depending upon the severity of the conjunctival response, staining and pooling may be visible. Sodium fluorescein pooling often will be seen outside the area directly affected by the contact lens and is associated with conjunctival chemosis. Circular conjunctival pooling will be evident if indentation has occurred. If epithelial damage has occurred, instillation of rose bengal and use of white light is the best method of detection.

Management

The management strategies for conjunctival trauma and hyperemia will vary according to the condition's severity. Contact lens wear sometimes causes small amounts of conjunctival staining and pooling, and it is often acceptable for patients with such findings to continue lens wear.

If severe hyperemia and staining are noted, however, a 1 to 7 day discontinuation may be needed. Therapeutic intervention may be necessary for some conjunctival complications, particularly if infection is suspected.[86] Antibiotics and patching may be necessary if the area of involvement is large or if the patient is experiencing discomfort[87] (see Figures 3-13 and 3-14).

Corneal Wrinkling

Etiology

Corneal wrinkling was first reported in 1987.[89] It occurs when (centrally) ultrathin lenses with excessively thick peripheries cause a "ripple" effect in the lens center.[89] Corneal wrinkling is probably caused by a combination of an inextensible lens periphery and such an excessively thin lens center that lid pressure cannot force the lens to conform to the eye, causing the lens to ripple. This rippling is then transferred to the cornea—perhaps as a result of a combination of pressure and dehydration (unpublished data).

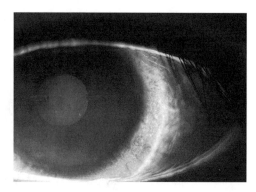

FIGURE 3-13 Soft contact lens edge-related staining.

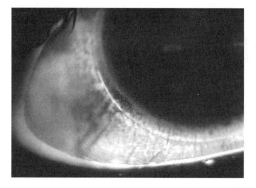

FIGURE 3-14 Conjunctival edge-related indentation pooling.

Signs and Symptoms

The corneal distortion associated with corneal wrinkling causes rapid and significant vision loss. A decrease from 6/6 to 6/60 acuity can occur within minutes of lens insertion.

Observation

The condition is easily observed using low magnification with sodium fluorescein and blue light.

Management

Corneal wrinkling is reversible. The time required for corneal distortion and subsequent vision loss to recover is approximately equal to the time the lens was worn before removal (unpublished data).

Corneal wrinkling may recur if the patient resumes wearing the same lens; the patient should therefore be refitted with a different lens design (see Figure 3-15).

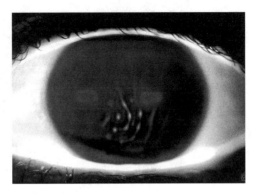

FIGURE 3-15 Typical fluorescein pooling in a case of epithelial winking.

Contact Lens Superior Limbic Keratoconjunctivitis (CLSLK)

Etiology

This multifactorial condition involves both the cornea and the conjunctiva. It is usually bilateral, but more advanced in one eye than the other. It is an uncommon condition and seems to occur only with hydrogel lens wear.[63,90,91]

Suspected causes of CLSLK are chronic hypoxia of corneal and conjunctival tissues under the upper lid, mechanical irritation from the lens edge moving over the limbus, and exposure to particular contact lens care preservatives, especially thimerosal.[90,91] It also has been suggested that CLSLK is an immunological response to antigens that deposit on the lens and is, in effect, an antibody-antigen reaction. Probably all of the above factors contribute, and care must be taken in treatment to account for all possible causes.[90,91]

Signs and Symptoms

Signs are superior limbic corneal and conjunctival hyperemia and fluorescein and rose bengal staining in the area of insertion of the superior rectus muscle. Epithelial haziness with underlying stromal infiltrates and micropannus also will be noted.[63,90,91]

Symptoms include decreased lens tolerance manifesting as lens awareness and decreased wearing time, burning and itching sensations, photophobia, and slight vision loss.[90,91]

Management

Symptoms generally resolve within 3 or 4 days of lens removal, although the signs may persist for several weeks. If symptoms persist, an ocular lubricant should be administered to minimize the mechanical insult the lid causes to the cornea and conjunctiva.[90]

When the condition has resolved and the inflammation subsided, an effective care regimen that excludes any thimerosal-preserved solutions should be used and an ocular lubricant prescribed.[90]

If the condition recurs, the practitioner should refit the patient with RGP lenses.

Superior Epithelial Arcuate Lesion (SEAL)

Etiology

Three hypotheses have been advanced regarding the etiology of superior epithelial arcuate lesion (SEAL) that, to date, has been reported only in patients wearing hydrogel lenses.[92] The first attributes the condition to mechanical chafing of the limbal area by a combination of pressures from the superior eyelid and the inner lens edge. The second suggests that hypoxia, exacerbated by the eyelid's position and pressure and the thickness of the lens edge contributes. The third hypothesis suggested is that of epithelial desiccation.[92]

Studies[92] show that the condition is more likely to occur in male presbyopes (where it affects both experienced and neophyte wearers) and in wearers of high water content lenses. Lens care regimen was not implicated in this analysis and they speculate that SEAL is caused by localized pressures that induce tear film thinning. It also was suggested that hypoxia and corneal fragility contribute to the condition.

Signs and Symptoms

SEAL is recognized by a characteristic band staining pattern and progresses through three stages:

1. Arcuate punctate staining
2. Coalesced punctate patches of damaged epithelium
3. An epithelial "split," sometimes full thickness, with a well-defined (0.5 mm wide) arcuate band of staining

No inflammation of the conjunctiva or limbus occurs, infiltrates are not present, and the upper lid is normal. The condition is generally asymptomatic and unilateral.

Observation

The condition is characteristically observed within 2 mm of the superior limbus in the area normally covered by the upper lid. It is only noted with the instillation of sodium fluorescein and diffuse blue light and can be seen with the Wratten #12 filter placed over the observation tube.

Management

Lens wear should be discontinued for a minimum of 1 week after which the lens, if in good condition, can be refitted. If the condition recurs, a 7-day discontinuation is recommended and the patient should then be fitted with lenses of a different design. It may be necessary to try a number of lens designs and materials before finding one that does not induce the condition. If soft lens alternatives fail to resolve the SEAL, the patient should be refitted with RGP lenses.[92]

Patient Management

We contend that extended wear of current hydrogel contact lenses is only acceptable for a minority of patients. It is therefore safer and in patients' long-term interests to remove lenses every night.

Daily wear of current hydrogel extended-wear lenses, combined with regular replacement, constitutes the safest and most successful form of contact lens wear today; however, if patient and practitioner persist with extended wear, patient education and compliance are extremely important.

Education

It is important with extended wear that the patient first demonstrate success and compliance on a daily-wear schedule. Before the decision is made to transfer the patient to extended wear, the onus is on the practitioner to educate the patient about possible long-term consequences.

Many aspects of lens wear need to be covered in patient education; if this is carried out thoroughly, both patient and practitioner will benefit. The patient should be instructed to regularly check the eye's redness, bulbar conjunctival comfort, vision, and lens mobility. By regularly monitoring these aspects of lens performance, the patient can then assess lens performance on waking and will be better able to detect any subtle changes following overnight wear.

The patient should be advised to use unit dose unpreserved saline as an in-eye solution before and after sleeping. This will rehydrate the lens and remove excess tear debris and mucous strands that might otherwise be a source of irritation.

The patient should be advised to remove the lenses if he or she notes any unusual lens or ocular response. The problem's severity will dictate the subsequent course of action. If the problem is minor, the patient should clean, rinse, and reinsert the lenses. However, if discomfort continues or ocular redness occurs after reinsertion, the patient should remove the lenses and immediately seek professional advice. Delay in seeking help can have serious consequences; this point must be repeatedly stressed.

CLINICAL PEARL

The patient should be advised to remove the lenses if he or she notes any unusual lens or ocular response.

The patient should be instructed to carefully assess the quality of his or her vision shortly after waking. Blurred vision that takes some time to clear (30 to 60 minutes after waking) may indicate excessive corneal edema. Overnight corneal edema may have disappeared by the time the patient is examined; any report from the patient of visual disturbance can assist the practitioner in determining the extended-wear performance of the patient's lenses.

Diminished vision on waking also may result from build-up of mucus and tear debris on or behind the lens. This is more likely to occur in extended wear's early stages; the patient should be made aware of excessive ocular discharge's effect on vision. If redness and discomfort are absent, the patient should instill unit dose saline onto the eye and lens and wipe away any ocular discharge from the upper and lower lid margins.

Extended wear patients must be informed that during periods of ill health they should not wear lenses on an extended-wear basis. Any debilitating illness can adversely affect the eye's ability to withstand the stress imposed on it by the overnight wear of contact lenses.

Aftercare Schedule

All contact lens patients should have regular eye examinations. The extended wear patient must be made to understand that frequent aftercare visits are important in determining his or her response to various factors and in the prevention of chronic effects that, in the majority of cases, would go undetected by the patient.

The successful extended-wear patient should see his or her clinician the day after fitting, and again after a week. Monthly visits should then be scheduled for the next 3 months, and for the remainder of the first year the patient should present for examination at 3 month intervals. After the first year, the patient must be examined on a quarterly basis.

Care and Maintenance

The recommended care schedule for hydrogel extended wear is to replace lenses weekly. If, however, this is impossible, the correct use of lens care products is essential. Thorough patient instruction in the recommended care and maintenance of lenses will promote compliance and minimize complications. Patients should be specifically instructed not to mix different brands of solutions. Care and maintenance of hydrogel extended-wear lenses must be specifically matched to the lens type and replacement schedule, as outlined in Table 3-6.

In summary, the patient should be instructed to observe the following steps:

1. Check regularly for ocular redness, satisfactory comfort and vision, and lens mobility in each eye.
2. Use unit dose unpreserved saline on waking and before sleep.
3. Remove the lenses if any irritation occurs, rinse with saline, and reinsert.
4. If irritation persists, the lens should be removed and the practitioner consulted.

TABLE 3-6

Care and Maintenance of Hydrogel Lenses

High Water Content	Low Water Content
Preferred Replacement Schedule	
Weekly removal and replacement	Weekly removal and replacement
Regular Replacement/Care Schedule	
Surfactant cleaner	Surfactant cleaner
Unpreserved saline rinse	Unpreserved saline rinse
Enzymatic cleaner (weekly)	Enzymatic cleaner (weekly)
Repeat surfactant cleaner	Repeat surfactant cleaner
Peroxide disinfection	Heat or peroxide disinfection
16-hour rest period	16-hour rest period

Conclusion

Our knowledge of the conditions that occur with the extended wear of hydrogel lenses and the appropriate practitioner response to them is incomplete. Other conditions may be encountered as extended wear is observed over a longer period. For example, we anticipate that chronic hypoxia with current hydrogel extended-wear lenses will lead to a significant incidence of compulsory discontinuation because of CES.

Disposable lenses reduce inflammatory response rates. In one study the contact lens acute red eye response rate was 4% for disposable mid water content lenses replaced every 1 or 2 weeks and 3% for regularly replaced low water content lenses.[48] This compares with a response rate of 34% in continuous-wear studies conducted in 1978[5] and 16% in later studies.[48] Furthermore, with regular replacement of both types of lenses, the incidence of CLPC is as low as 3% annually.[48]

The introduction of simpler one-step care systems also can improve patient compliance. The new generation of enzymatic cleaners now becoming available offers simplified lens care that should further improve compliance. The development of lens surfaces that reduce adherence of protein deposits and encourage their effective removal by the care system also will enhance the safety and clinical success of hydrogel extended wear.

The decrease in adverse response rates with disposable lenses has not yet been matched by improved physiological performance with hydrogel extended wear. Overnight edema, microcysts, and polymegethism are still the norm. Until hydrogel lenses offering greater oxygen transmissibility become available, a reduction in the number of nights of lens wear per week is the only means available to prevent chronic hypoxia. It remains to be seen whether advances in materials and lens care will allow wear schedules to more closely approach ideal levels for patient convenience.

References

1. De Carle J: Developing hydrophilic lenses for continuous wearing, *Aust J Optom* 55:343-346, 1972.
2. Weissman BA: An introduction to extended wear contact lenses, *J Am Optom Assoc* 53:183-186, 1982.
3. Schwartz CA: Contact lens update 1986, *Cont Lens Forum* 11(1):23-59, 1986.
4. Ruben M, Brown N, Lobascher D, Chaston J, Morris J: Clinical manifestations secondary to soft lens wear, *Br J Ophthalmol* 60:529-530, 1976.
5. Zantos SG, Holden BA: Ocular changes associated with continuous wear of contact lenses, *Aust J Optom* 61:418-426, 1978.
6. Mondino BJ, Weissman BJ, Farb MD, Pettit TH: Corneal ulcers associated with daily wear and extended wear contact lenses, *Am J Ophthalmol* 102:58-65, 1986.
7. Chalupa E, Swarbrick HA, Holden BA, Sjostrand J: Severe corneal infections associated with contact lens wear, *Ophthalmol* 94:17-22, 1987.
8. Cooper RL, Constable IJ: Infective keratitis in soft contact lens wearers, *Br J Ophthalmol* 61:250-254, 1977.
9. Schein OD, Glynn RJ, Poggio EC, Seddon JM, Kenyon KR, and the Microbial Keratitis Study Group: The relative risk of ulcerative keratitis among users of daily-wear and extended wear soft contact lenses, *N Engl J Med* 321:773-778, 1989.
10. Poggio EC, Glynn RJ, Schein OD, Seddon JM, Shannon MJ, Scardino VA, Kenyon KR: The incidence of ulcerative keratitis among users of daily wear and extended wear soft contact lenses, *N Eng J Med* 321:779-783, 1989.
11. Lippman RE: The FDA role in contact lens development and safety, *Cornea* 9 (Suppl 1) S64-S68, 1990.
12. FDA Practitioner Letter: Ulcerative keratitis and contact lens wear, May 30, 1989.
13. Mertz GW: Overnight swelling of the living human cornea, *J Am Optom Assoc* 51:211-214, 1980.
14. Holden BA, Mertz GW, McNally JJ: Corneal swelling response to contact lenses worn under extended wear conditions, *Inv Ophthalmol Vis Sci* 24:218-226, 1983.
15. La Hood D, Sweeney DF, Holden BA: Overnight corneal edema with hydrogel rigid gas permeable and silicone elastomer contact lenses, *Int Cont Lens Clin* 15:149-153, 1988.
16. Efron N, Holden BA: A review of some common contact lens complications. Part 1: The corneal epithelium and stroma, *Optician* 192 (5057):21-26, 1986.
17. Holden BA, Sweeney DF, Vannas A, Nilsson KT, Efron N: Effects of long-term extended contact lens wear on the human cornea, *Inv Ophthalmol Vis Sci* 26:1489-1501, 1985.
18. Madigan MC, Holden BA, Kwok LS: Extended wear of contact lenses can compromise corneal epithelial adhesion, *Curr Eye Res* 6:1257-1260, 1987.
19. La Hood D, Grant T, Holden BA: Characteristics of overnight corneal edema responses caused by RGP and soft contact lenses, *Am J Optom Physiol Opt* 64:99, 1987.
20. Efron N: Clinical management of corneal edema, *Cont Lens Spec* 1(12);13-23, 1986.
21. Holden BA: The Glenn A Fry Award Lecture 1988. The ocular response to contact lens wear, *Optom Vis Sci* 66(11):717-733, 1989.
22. Madigan M: Animal models for extended wear contact lenses, PhD thesis, University of New South Wales, Sydney, Australia, 1990.
23. Holden BA, Grant T, Kotow M, Schnider C, Sweeney DF: Epithelial microcysts with daily and extended wear of hydrogel and rigid gas-permeable contact lenses, *Inv Ophthalmol Vis Sci* 28 (Suppl): 372, 1987.
24. Zantos SG: Cystic formations in the corneal epithelium during extended wear of contact lenses, *Int Cont Lens Clin* 10(3):128-146, 1983.
25. Terry RL, Schnider CM, Holden BA, Cornish R, Grant T, Sweeney D, La Hood D, Back A. CCLRU standards for success of daily and extended wear contact lenses, *Optom Vis Sci* 70(3):234-243, 1993.

26. Schoessler JP, Woloschak M: Corneal endothelium in veteran PMMA contact lens wearers, *Int Cont Lens Clin* 8:19-25, 1981.

27. Caldwell DR, Kastri PR, Dabezies OH, Kirby R, Miller BS, Hawk TJ: The effect of long-term hard lens wear on corneal endothelium, *Cont Lens* 8 (2) 87-91, 1982.

28. Schoessler JP: Corneal endothelial polymegethism associated with extended wear, *Int Cont Lens Clinic* 10:148-155, 1983.

29. Stocker EG, Schoessler JP: Corneal endothelial polymegethism induced by PMMA contact lens wear, *Inv Ophthalmol Vis Sci* 26(6):857-863, 1985.

30. MacRae SM, Matsuda M, Yee R: The effect of long-term hard contact lens wear on the corneal endothelium, *CLAO* 11(4):322-326, 1985.

31. Conner C, Zagrod M: Contact-lens induced corneal endothelial polymegethism: functional significance and possible mechanisms, *Am J Optom Physiol Opt* 63(7):539-544, 1986.

32. Bonanno JA, Polse KA: Corneal acidosis during contact lens wear: effects of hypoxia and CO_2, *Inv Ophthalmol Vis Sci* 28:1514-1520, 1987.

33. Sweeney DF, Holden BA, Vannas A, Efron N, Swarbrick H, Kotow M, Chan-Ling T: The clinical significance of corneal endothelial polymegethism, *Inv Ophthalmol Vis Sci* 26 (Suppl):53, 1985.

34. Polse KA, Brand RJ, Cohen SR, Guillon M: Hypoxic effects on corneal morphology and function, *Inv Ophthalmol Vis Sci* 31 (4) Suppl. 2000, 1990.

35. Holden BA, Vannas A, Nilsson K, Efron N, Sweeney D, Kotow M, La Hood D, Guillon M: Epithelial and endothelial effects from the extended wear of contact lenses, *Curr Eye Res* 4:739-742, 1985.

36. Zantos SG, Holden BA: Transient endothelial changes soon after wearing soft contact lenses, *Am J Optom Physiol Opt* 54:856-858, 1977.

37. Holden BA, Williams L, Zantos SG: The etiology of transient endothelial changes in the human cornea, *Inv Ophthalmol Vis Sci* 26(10): 1354, 1985.

38. Vannas A, Holden BA, Makitie J: The ultrastructure of contact lens induced changes, *Acta Ophthalmol* 62:320-333, 1984.

39. Williams L, Holden BA: The bleb response of the endothelium decreases with extended wear of contact lenses, *Clin Exp Optom* 69:90-92, 1986.

40. Holden BA, Sweeney DF: Corneal Exhaustion Syndrome (CES) in long-term contact lens wearers - A consequence of contact lens-induced polymegethism?, *Am J Optom Physiol Opt* 65:95P, 1988.

41. Back AP: Corneal staining with contact lens wear, *Trans BCLA* 5 16-18, 1988.

42. Efron N: Management of ocular complications of contact lens wear: A systematic approach, *BCLA Scientific Meetings* 32-34, 1988.

43. McMonnies CW, Zantos SG: Endothelial bedewing of the cornea in association with contact lens wear, *Br J Ophthalmol* 62:478, 1981.

44. Josephson JE, Caffery BE: Infiltrative keratitis in hydrogel lens wearers, *Int Cont Lens Clin* 6:223-242, 1979.

45. Zantos SG: The ocular response to continuous wear of contact lenses. PhD Thesis, University of NSW, Sydney, Australia, 1981.

46. Zantos SG: Management of corneal infiltrates in extended wear contact lens patients, *Int Cont Lens Clin* 11:604-610, 1984.

47. Gordon A, Kracher GP: Corneal infiltrates and extended wear lenses, *J Am Optom Assoc* 56(3) 198-201, 1985.

48. Grant T, Chong MS, Holden BA: Which is best for the eye: daily wear, 2 night or 6 nights, *Am J Optom Physiol Opt* 65(10) Suppl 40p, 1988.

49. Mertz GW, Holden BA: Clinical implications of extended wear research, *Can J Optom* 43:203-205, 1981.

50. Holden BA, La Hood D, Grant T, Newton-Howes J, Baleriola-Lucas C, Willcox M, Sweeney D: Gram-negative can induce contact lens related acute red eye (CLARE) responses, (In preparation).

51. Kotow M, Grant T, Holden BA: Avoiding ocular complications during hydrogel extended wear, *Int Cont Lens Clin* 14:95-99, 1987.

52. Newton-Howes J, Durany N, Grant T, Holden BA: The distribution of proteins on the surface and in the matrix of hydrogel contact lenses, *Optom Vis Sci* 66 (10) Suppl: 90, 1989.

53. Burnett-Hodd NF: Some observations on 62 permanent wear soft lens cases, *Ophthalmic Optician* 3-8, Nov 15, 1975.

54. Nilsson SEG, Montan PG: The hospitalized cases of contact lens induced keratitis in Sweden and their relation to lens type and wear schedule: results of a three-year retrospective study, *CLAO* 20(2):97-101, 1994.

55. Grant T, Chong MS, Fleming C, Swarbrick H, Gauthier C, Sweeney D, Holden BA: Culture negative peripherial ulcers (CNPU) during hydrogel contact lens wear, (Submitted for publication-*CLAO*).

56. Hyndiuk RA, Nassif KF, Burd EM: Infectious diseases. In Smolin G, Thoft RA (eds): *The cornea: scientific foundations & clinical practice*, Boston, 1983, Little Brown & Co., 147-167.

57. Adams CP, Cohen EJ, Laibson PR, Galentine P, Arentsen JJ: Corneal ulcers in patients with cosmetic extended-wear contact lenses, *Am J Ophthalmol* 96:705-709, 1983.

58. Galentine PG, Cohen EJ, Laibson PR, Adams CP, Michaud R, Arentsen JJ: Corneal ulcers associated with contact lens wear, *Arch Ophthalmol* 102:891-894, 1984.

59. Lemp MA, Blackman HJ, Wilson CA, Leveille AS: Gram-negative corneal ulcers in elderly aphakic eyes with extended-wear lenses, *Ophthalmol* 91:60-63, 1984.

60. Spoor TC, Hartel WC, Wynn P, Spoor DK: Complications of continuous wear soft contact lenses in a non-referral population, *Arch Ophthalmol* 102:1312-1313, 1984.

61. Leisegang TJ, Forster RK: Spectrum of microbial keratitis in south Florida, *Am J Ophthalmol* 90:38-47, 1980.

62. Eichenbaum JW, Feldstein M, Podos SM: Extended-wear aphakic soft contact lenses and corneal ulcers, *Br J Ophthalmol* 66:663-666, 1982.

63. Catania LJ: *Primary care of the anterior segment*, East Norwalk, 1988, Appleton & Lange.

64. Wallace W: Soft contact lens associated infectious corneal ulcer, *Int Eyecare* 2(3):171-172, 1986.

65. Spring TF: Reactions to hydrophilic lenses, *Med J Aust* 1:449-450, 1974.

66. Allansmith MR, Korb DR, Greiner JV, Henriquez AS, Simon MA, Finnemore VM: Giant papillary conjunctivitis in contact lens wearers, *Am J Ophthalmol* 83:697-708, 1977.

67. Barishak Y, Zavaro A, Samra Z, Sompolinsky D: An immunologic study of papillary conjunctivitis due to contact lenses, *Curr Eye Res* 3:1161-1168, 1984.

68. Herman JP: Clinical management of GPC, *Cont Lens Spectrum* 2 (11):24-36, 1987.

69. Molinari JF: The clinical management of giant papillary conjunctivitis, *Am J Optom Physiol Opt* 58:886-891, 1981.

70. Molinari JF: Review: giant papillary conjunctivitis, *Aust J Optom* 66:59-67, 1983.

71. Fowler SA, Greiner JV, Allansmith MR: Soft contact lenses from patients with giant papillary conjunctivitis, *Am J Ophthalmol* 88:1056-1061, 1979.

72. Grant T, Holden BA, Rechberger J, Chong MS: Contact lens related papillary conjunctivitis (CLRPC): influence of protein accumulation and replacement frequency, *Inv Ophthalmol Vis Sci* 30 (3) Suppl. 166, 1989.

73. Grant T, Chong MS, Holden BA: Management of GPC with daily disposable lenses, *Am J Optom Physiol Opt* 65:(10) Suppl:94P, 1988.

74. Herman JP: Clinical management of GPC, *Cont Lens Spectrum* 2:(12) 41-43, 1987.

75. Donshik PC, Ballow M, Luistro A, Samartino L: Treatment of contact lens-induced giant papillary conjunctivitis, *CLAO* 10:346-350, 1984.

76. Molinari JF, Rengstorff R: Management of soft lens-induced GPC with vitamin A aqueous drops, *Cont Lens* 16:(7):169-170, 1988.

77. Fromer CH, Klintworth GK: An evaluation of the role of leukocytes in the pathogenesis of experimentally induced corneal vascularization. III. Studies related to the vasoproliferative capability of polymorphonuclear leukocytes and lymphocytes, *Am J Pathol* 82:157-167, 1976.

78. Imre G: Vascularization of the eye. In Bellows JG (ed.): *Contemporary Ophthalmology*, Baltimore, 1972, Williams and Wilkins, 88-91.

79. McMonnies CW: Risk factors in the etiology of contact lens-induced corneal vascularization, *Int Cont Lens Clin* 11:286-293, 1984.

80. McMonnies CW: Contact lens-induced corneal vascularization, *Int Cont Lens Clin* 10(1):12-21, 1983.

81. McMonnies CW, Chapman-Davies A, Holden BA: The vascular response to contact lens wear, *Am J Optom Physiol Opt* 59:795-799, 1982.

82. Kame RT: Adverse ocular response to soft lens solutions, *Cont Lens Forum* 9(1):97-101, 1984.

83. Cioletti KR: Determination of thimerosal content in contact lens polymers, *Int Cont Lens Clin* 7:16-20, 1980.

84. Mondino BJ, Groden LR: Conjunctival hyperemia and corneal infiltrates with chemically disinfected soft contact lenses, *Arch Ophthalmol* 98(10):1767-1777, 1980.

85. Ruben CM: Contact lens solutions and allergic, toxic and inflammatory reactions, *Cont Lens* 15(3):8, 1987.

86. Brennan NA: Current thoughts on the etiology of ocular changes during contact lens wear, *Aust J Optom* 68(1):8-24, 1985.

87. Locke LC: Conjunctival abrasions and lacerations, *J Am Optom Assoc* 58(6):488-493, 1987.

88. McMonnies CW: After-care symptoms, signs and management. In Phillips AJ, Stone J (eds.): *Contact lenses: a textbook for practitioner and student*, London, 1989, Butterworths, 703-736.

89. Lowe R, Brennan NA: Corneal wrinkling caused by a thin medium water contact lens, *Int Cont Lens Clin* 14(10):403-406, 1987.

90. Abel R, Shovlin JP, DePaolis MD: A treatise on hydrophilic lens induced superior limbic keratoconjunctivitis, *Int Cont Lens Clin* 12(2):116-123, 1985.

91. Sendele DD, Kenyon KR, Mobila EF, Rosenthal P, Steinert R, Hanninen LA: Superior limbic keratoconjunctivitis in contact lens wearers, *Ophthalmol* 90(6):616-622, 1983.

92. Hine NA, Back AP, Holden BA: Aetiology of arcuate epithelial lesions induced by hydrogels, *Trans BCLA* 4:48-50, 1984.

4

Rigid Gas-Permeable Extended Wear

Kenneth A. Polse
Reuben K. Rivera
Cheslyn M. Gan

Key Terms

rigid gas-permeable extended wear lenses	endothelial polymegethism	lens adhesion oxygen transmissibility
corneal edema	superficial punctate keratitis	
epithelial microcysts	corneal acidosis	

Complications of rigid gas-permeable extended wear (RGPEW) can be divided into two areas, those resulting from metabolic interruptions to normal corneal physiology and those resulting from mechanical insult. Complications from metabolic disturbance include corneal edema, epithelial microcysts, endothelial polymegethism, and superficial punctate keratitis (SPK). Mechanical changes accompanying RGPEW include temporal and nasal SPK (3-9 o'clock limbal staining) and lens adherence.

These physiological disturbances primarily result from altered epithelial metabolism. Most current research indicates that if the cornea is exposed to a hypoxic environment normal metabolism is affected, causing a movement of lactate into the corneal stroma. This results in a reduction in pH and an increased osmotic load, leading to stromal edema.[1] The decrease in corneal pH (corneal acidosis) alters the extracellular fluid surrounding the epithelial and endothelial cells, resulting in changes in the morphology and physiology of these two layers. Corneal acidosis can be prevented if sufficient oxygen levels are present to prevent the cornea from shifting to anaerobic metabolism.[2]

In addition to corneal hypoxia, the tissue's pH can be reduced if a build-up of carbon dioxide (CO_2) occurs between the contact lens and cornea. This CO_2-induced pH drop occurs when the eyes are closed, whether or not a contact lens is worn. If a contact lens does not adequately pump fluid when the eye is open, CO_2 will remain trapped behind the lens. This allows the decrease in pH to continue during the open-eye condition. However, most gas-permeable rigid contact lenses provide sufficient tear pumping so that the CO_2 build-up from sleep is quickly depleted after the eye opens and normal tear pumping resumes. Also, the rigid lens provides for carbon dioxide transmissibility (Dk CO_2/L) so that some carbon dioxide is removed directly through the lens itself. This combination of carbon dioxide lens transmission and good tear pumping prevents any change in pH with rigid lenses when the eyes are open.

It is apparent from clinical examination that corneas exposed to chronic hypoxia will have stromal edema, microcysts, polymegethism, and superficial punctate keratitis.[3-9] These metabolic complications should be identified and appropriately managed regardless of the exact mechanism.

Physiological Complications

Corneal edema is the classic sign of hypoxia and should alert the clinician to the possible development of other metabolically related problems. It is best observed using the slit lamp biomicroscope in a completely dark room with the observer partially dark adapted. The best slit lamp technique is indirect retroillumination. Because edema from contact lens wear subsides rapidly, it is best observed within an hour after the patient wakes. Indeed, observations 3 to 4 hours after eye opening will usually show no corneal edema, even in patients with a severe overnight edematous response.

CLINICAL PEARL

Corneal edema is the classic sign of hypoxia and should alert the clinician to the possible development of other metabolically related problems.

Vertical lines (corneal striae) usually accompany edema in the posterior cornea.[10,11] These lines usually are seen when the cornea has developed 6% or greater edema.[10,11] As edema increases, the number and density of the striae also increase. Because striae are relatively easy to observe, identification of these lines should be part of evaluating an edematous response. Striae can be graded on a 0 to 3 scale, where grade 0 indicates no striae, grade 1 indicates 1 or 2 faint lines, grade 2 indicates 2 to 6 lines, and grade 3 indicates many lines along with black folds easily observed with the slit lamp.

Most currently approved RGPEW lenses cause corneal edema when worn with the eyes closed (e.g., during sleep). The edema pattern is illustrated in Figure 4-1, which shows an increase in edema during the closed-eye period but a relatively rapid recovery once the eyes are open. The edematous pattern occurs each day the lenses are worn on an extended-wear schedule.[12] Figure 4-1 also shows that most of the edema subsides two hours after the eye opens. The clinician must see the patient soon after eye opening to observe edema. This is usually difficult to manage and most of the edema will go undetected by the clinician.

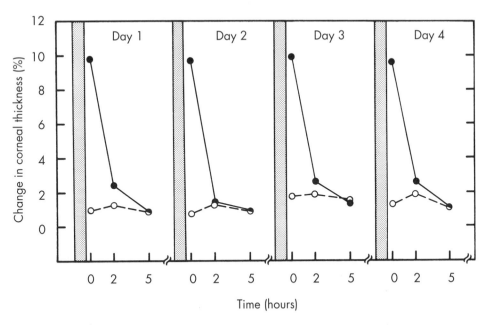

FIGURE 4-1 Mean corneal thickness changes over a 4-day period of wear of hard gas-permeable extended-wear lenses. Filled circles indicate the test eye wearing the lens on an extended-wear basis; open circles indicate the control eye wearing the lens on a daily-wear basis. Time is measured from opening of the test eye. (From Kenyon E, Polse KA, O'Neal MD: Ocular response to extended wear of hard gas-permeable lenses, *CLAO* 11:119-123, 1985.)

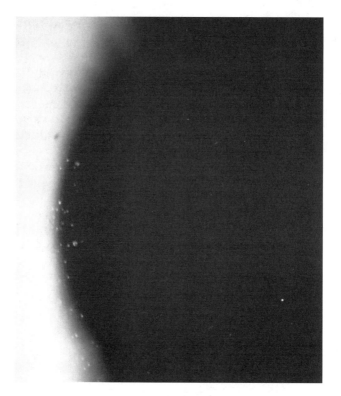

FIGURE 4-2 Microcysts. (Courtesy of Dr. Emily Kenyon.)

The clinician should therefore rely on patient symptoms such as blurred or variable vision in the morning, photophobia, and minor discomfort upon waking. If these symptoms are present, the clinician should suspect edema and try to examine the patient early in the morning. In any case regular follow-up examinations are necessary to monitor and care for the possible development of microcysts and polymegethism.

Epithelial microcysts were first reported in soft lens extended wear (Figure 4-2).[9,13] More recently they have been reported with most RGPEW materials.[14] These cysts usually take 2 or 3 months to occur, begin at the deeper epithelial layers, and migrate anteriorly. If they reach the surface, they cause a break in the epithelium that will stain with fluorescein dye. It has been suggested that the microcysts be counted; however, we have not found this practical and recommend a grading system based on the density and presence or absence of epithelial staining.[15] Figure 4-3 shows the recommended grading system for microcystic response.

Microcysts are clinically important because they represent a change in the epithelial tissue's morphology and physiology. Thus the epithelium's normal protective function may be altered and the opportunity

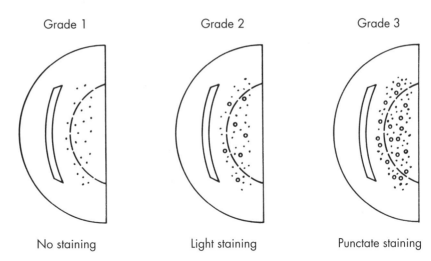

FIGURE 4-3 Microcyst grading system. Because microcysts quickly develop to a point where they can no longer be accurately counted, a grading system based on density was devised. Higher grades of microcysts are frequently accompanied by light punctate keratitis; when more than two microcysts stained, they were given a minimum of grade 2. (From Kenyon E, Polse KA, Seger RG: Influence of wearing schedule on extended-wear complications, *Ophthalmol* 93:231-236, 1986.)

for infection may be greater than when microcysts are absent. The microcystic response tends to be chronic, and even if contact lens wear is discontinued it may take several weeks or months to resolve. We recommend that patients who show a grade 2 or greater microcystic response return to daily wear. In our experience, remission of the microcysts with gas-permeable daily wear is equivalent to the patient discontinuing lens wear altogether. It is therefore unnecessary for the patient to discontinue all lens wear, just the overnight cycle.

CLINICAL PEARL

Microcysts are clinically important because they represent a change in the epithelial tissue's morphology and physiology.

After the microcysts have resolved, the patient may go back to extended wear if a new lens with a higher oxygen transmissibility is available. If such a lens is unavailable, we recommend that the patient continue with daily wear until a high Dk material can be fitted.

Disturbed physiology also causes morphological changes in the corneal endothelium.[16] These changes result primarily in disturbance

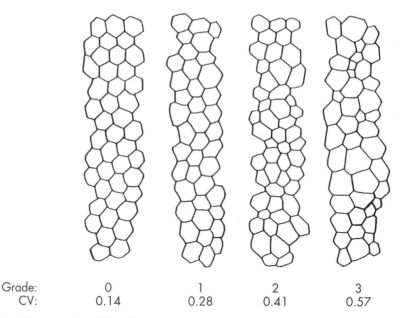

Grade:	0	1	2	3
CV:	0.14	0.28	0.41	0.57

FIGURE 4-4 The CCLRU polymegethism grading system. (Courtesy of Dr. Brien A. Holden, Cornea and Contact Lens Research Unit at the University of New South Wales.)

of the uniform hexagonal pattern seen in most normal endothelial cell layers. Over a period of months to years the endothelium becomes irregular in cell size and shape. This condition is called polymegethism. Occasionally, irregularity and loss of hexagonality accompany extended wear. This condition is called pleomorphism. The effect of contact–lens-induced morphological changes is not well understood. Because the endothelium is the primary site for maintaining normal corneal hydration, the clinician should exercise concern and some conservatism when changes are seen.

We recommend using a endothelial grading system based on one initially suggested by Holden et al[17] (Figure 4-4). The amount of polymegethism displayed by the endothelial mosaic is graded on a 0 to 3 scale, where 0 represents no morphological changes, and grades 1, 2, and 3 represent slight, moderate, and marked polymegethism, respectively. The numerical values shown in Figure 4-4 represent the coefficient of variation in endothelial cell size. The value is defined as the standard deviation of cell area divided by the mean cell area.

Figure 4-5 shows the endothelial mosaic of a 75-year-old patient with a normal cornea, the normal endothelial mosaic of a 25-year-old nonwearer, and the endothelium of a 25-year-old patient who has worn extended-wear lenses for 3 years. The striking similarity between the extended-wear patient and the older patient allows one to hypothesize that contact lens extended wear changes

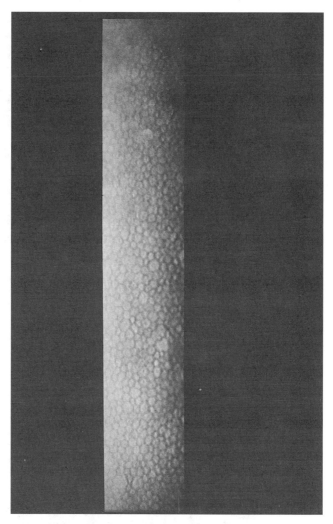

FIGURE 4-5 A, Normal endothelial mosaic of a 75-year-old non–contact-lens wearer.   *Continued*

the morphology in a "premature aging" fashion. This change's etiology seems to be prolonged corneal hypoxia. Moderate or marked polymegethism should be dealt with by having the patient return to daily wear or be fitted with a lens of much higher oxygen transmissibility.

Hypoxic contact lens wear can permanently alter corneal function. Using a test that measures the rate at which the cornea recovers from induced edema, investigators found that patients with long-term PMMA experience showed slower recovery rates (expressed as percent recovery per hour or PRPH) compared to nonwearers.[18] Presumably

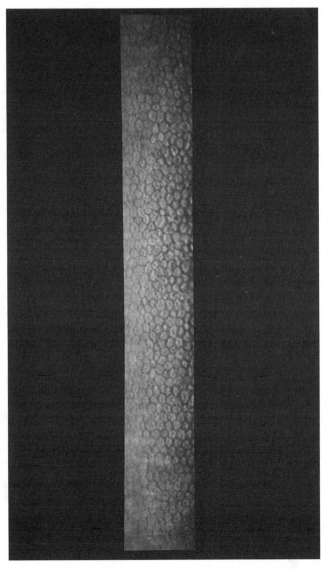

FIGURE 4-5, cont'd B, Normal endothelial mosaic of a 25-year-old non–contact-lens wearer.

this reduction in PRPH was permanent, apparently related to the number of years of lens wear, and caused by chronic hypoxia.[18] Other studies suggest a relationship between cell morphology and PRPH; increased endothelial polymegethism is associated with decreased PRPH. This finding would be consistent with the observed increase in polymegethism and decreased function that has been independently reported in long-term PMMA wearers.

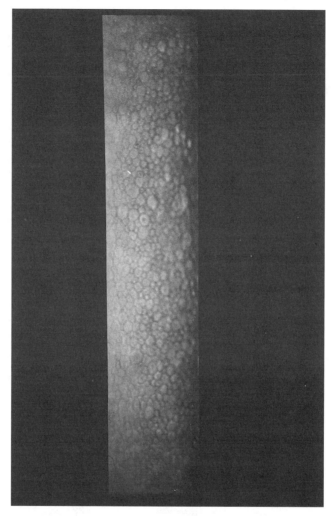

FIGURE 4-5, cont'd   C, Endothelial mosaic of a 25-year-old who has worn contact lenses on a extended-wear basis for 3 years.

Metabolic disturbances resulting from RGPEW also can lead to epithelial cell loss, usually observed as pinpoint staining. However, if the metabolic insult is severe enough, punctate staining also may be present. Usually, substantial hypoxia is required to produce punctate staining; however, even in patients who show a grade 2 microcystic response punctate staining may be present. In the presence of epithelial staining, the patient should resume daily contact lens wear, because epithelial cell loss may put the patient at risk for microbial keratitis.

The complications discussed above result from corneal hypoxia. We have had the opportunity to study the prevalence of these complications in patients whom we have fitted with RGPEW lenses. We have been able to fit many of these patients with improved oxygen-permeable material and have observed relative reductions in complications. This has provided us with important information concerning the mechanisms of these complications.

These complications are driven by insufficient oxygen[6,14,19-21] and more importantly from a clinical management viewpoint, they can be reduced or eliminated with appropriate oxygen levels. Figures 4-6 and 4-7 show the relative frequencies and amounts of corneal edema and microcysts occurring with lenses of various oxygen transmissibilities. Lenses with transmissibilities in the mid-40 range produce little adverse ocular response. For patients with moderate oxygen requirements, these lenses may be feasible for extended wear. Undoubtedly, the new generation of RGPEW materials with transmissibilities of $70\times$ to 80×10^{-9} (cm $\times$ ml $\times$ O_2)/(sec $\times$ ml $\times$ mm Hg) or greater will satisfy closed-eye metabolic requirements.[20] We should not get metabolic insult when patients use these lenses for extended wear. This does not imply that the new high Dk materials are necessarily safe. As we shall discuss, there are two mechanical problems unrelated to metabolic mechanisms that could limit RGPEW's success.

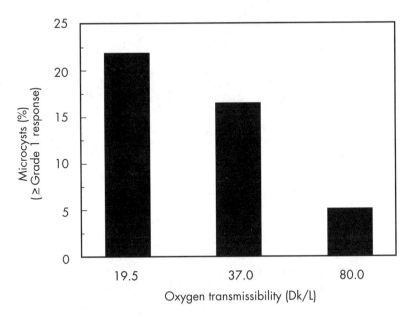

FIGURE 4-6 Relative frequencies of microcysts accompanying lenses of various oxygen transmissibilities. The frequency of this complication indicates at least a grade 1 or greater response after 6 months of rigid gas-permeable extended wear.

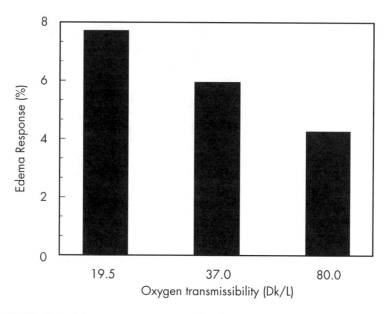

FIGURE 4-7 Mean percent corneal edema response accompanying lenses of various oxygen transmissibilities worn on an extended-wear basis.

Mechanical Complications

Mechanical complications related to RGPEW include lens binding, adherence, nasal/temporal superficial punctate keratitis (SPK), and 3-9 o'clock limbal staining. Adherence occurs when the contact lens binds to the cornea after the eyes are opened following a period of eye closure, causing SPK and corneal distortion (see Figure 4-8). If lens adherence occurs on a regular basis, it may lead to ulceration[22,23] or prolonged corneal distortion with spectacle blur.

The adherent lens is usually located at a peripheral corneal position, often without its edge crossing the limbus. Under the lens' midperiphery the tear film often appears foamy.[24,25] When fluorescein is instilled, it does not penetrate the foamy area. If adherence is weak, lens movement may begin after a few blinks. More often, however, it takes minutes or occasionally hours for the lens to resume normal movement if no force is applied to the lens. In all cases lens adherence is easily broken by manipulating the lens with the lids. When the lens is removed, a superficial punctate keratitis is usually found, especially in the area where foam had been observed. In addition, the adherent lens' pressure leaves an indentation in the cornea at the lens edge or peripheral curve junction.[24,25] This frequently causes corneal distortion, particularly in the area where the lens adhered.

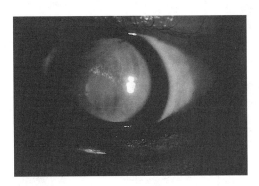

FIGURE 4-8 Rigid lens adherence staining seen after lens removal. (Courtesy of Dr. Cheslyn Gan.)

A number of factors interact to cause this phenomenon. Lens adhesion during RGPEW may result from lens decentration during the closed-eye state. During sleep an increase in tear viscosity reduces the lens' chance to recenter itself onto the central cornea. Lid pressure on the lens then creates a negative pressure that holds the lens on the flatter corneal periphery and limbus.[26,27] Finally, lens binding may result from the loss of the tears' aqueous portion during sleep, leaving the mucin layer to bind with the surface epithelium. Because dry eye patients often experience lens binding during open-eye wear, this mechanism during sleep seems possible. Therefore, when lens adherence accompanying closed-eye wear is suspected, a careful work-up for dry eye should be completed.

Rigid lens parameters can be altered to eliminate or reduce lens adhesion.[27-29] The lens modifications recommended by a number of studies have been contradictory at times and the question of how to counteract this phenomenon is unanswered.[27-29] Adhesion can be minimized in some patients by initially fitting RGPEW lenses with an alignment or slightly flat bearing relationship with the cornea. If adhesion occurs, refitting with a flatter back optic zone radius (BOZR), a smaller back optic zone diameter (BOZD), and a flatter peripheral system may help ease the problem.[27]

Rigid lens adherence often goes undetected by clinician and patient and has few immediate sequelae, except for corneal distortion, which may affect spectacle vision for a considerable length of time. Unless patients can detect the adherence themselves, practitioners cannot be sure of the diagnosis without examining the patients soon after sleep to detect the characteristic biomicroscopic signs. Because patients often cannot be examined upon waking, data are needed on the appearance and rapidity of corneal recovery to help clinicians make decisions regarding patient management.

The major concern about rigid lens adherence is induced epithelial breakdown.[24] Whenever a break occurs in the integrity of the corneal epithelium, the risk of infection increases, and early diagnosis is critical. There have been at least two reports of corneal ulcers caused by rigid lens adherence.[24,25] Thus although rigid extended-wear lenses generally produce fewer and milder adverse effects,[30,31] adherence is one adverse effect that is more serious with rigid extended wear than with soft lens extended wear.

CLINICAL PEARL

The major concern about rigid lens adherence is induced epithelial breakdown. Whenever a break occurs in the integrity of the corneal epithelium, the risk of infection increases, and early diagnosis is critical.

The second concern with rigid lens adherence is corneal distortion. In our studies distortion caused by rigid lens adherence was more frequent and severe than that caused by soft lens adherence. The keratometry mires after rigid lens adherence are typically distorted in one sector, corresponding to the corneal area in which the compression ring is seen with the biomicroscope. Temporary and minor distortion in an extended-wear contact lens patient is only of minor concern. However, it is our clinical impression that when the distortion is more severe it also is more prolonged.[24] Some patients with persistent rigid lens adherence show distorted mires even at the end of a day of contact lens wear or after a night without lenses. Previous experience with PMMA lenses showed that corneal distortion induced under hypoxic conditions could last for months, and in some cases appeared permanent.[32] For this reason, keratometry should be performed at every visit and overnight wear should be discontinued if distortion is seen on several visits.

We found that extended-wear rigid lens adherence has a higher incidence than has previously been reported, and that adherence occurs with soft extended-wear lenses and with rigid lenses. In the rigid–lens-wearing eye, 48% of subjects had biomicroscopic signs indicative of lens adherence. Of these subjects, 32% had observed adherence upon examination.[24]

The diagnosis of adherence can be difficult when it is not observed directly. The presence of SPK or corneal distortion is not diagnostic of this condition. Diagnosis depends upon observation of ringlike corneal indentation or characteristic arcuate staining.

Indentation often disappears within an hour after the lens begins to move.[24] Corneal staining also recovers quickly, and within an hour the characteristic arcuate-pattern SPK may become indistinguishable from SPK not caused by adherence. Thus the practitioner should see the patient as soon as possible after waking to determine whether adherence occurs. Our experience shows that even with early observation, patients with a history of rigid lens adherence will not show signs of adherence every day.

The practitioner should schedule the first two or three visits as early in the morning as possible. In practice, it is usually not feasible for patients to be examined just after sleep. Therefore, even patients who can be examined early should be instructed to look for the following signs of lens adherence upon waking:

1. A nonmoving lens
2. Blurred vision
3. Spectacle blur
4. Dry, gritty lenses or discharge
5. Conjunctival injection that subsides during the day

To observe their lenses, patients should look at their eyes in the mirror with adequate light between themselves and the mirror. If they have trouble seeing the lenses, marking dots can be placed on them for better visibility. Patients may choose to have a family member check the lenses. None of the symptoms listed above except lack of lens movement is necessarily diagnostic, but if patients report several symptoms the practitioner must consider the possibility of lens adherence.

Limbal staining has been observed and exhaustively studied during the period in which PMMA wear was popular. Limbal staining accompanying hard lens wear has been a clinical problem for about 10% to 15% of all hard lens wearers. The introduction of gas-permeable material has not altered this problem's incidence. If limbal staining is severe and not treated, the peripheral cornea may undergo several changes. Figure 4-9 shows an RGP wearer who has developed basement membrane thickening, neovascularization, SPK, conjunctival hyperemia, and extreme irregularity of the superficial epithelium as a result of limbal staining. In some cases drying can cause marked dellen formation. Although Figure 4-9 represents an extreme complication of limbal staining, chronic abuse to the peripheral cornea can result in these kinds of changes.

Many theories relating to limbal SPK's etiology have been set forth. Perhaps the most plausible suggests that limbal SPK results from drying of the peripheral cornea during contact lens wear. Indeed, patients with borderline dry eye will tend to show limbal staining. These factors also may contribute to or aggravate limbal staining.

Other factors include low-riding lenses, lenses that move too quickly inferiorly or temporally, lenses with excessively thick edges, or thick lenses (> .20 mm) that may produce lid gap and allow the area between the edge and the conjunctiva to dry out. If all these factors are eliminated and the lens appears to ride appropriately, 3-9 o'clock staining is probably related to dry eye, and tests to rule out this diagnosis should be done. Tests of aqueous, mucin, and lipid components, along with a careful inspection for surface abnormalities and epitheliopathies, need to be done. If dry eye is confirmed, the

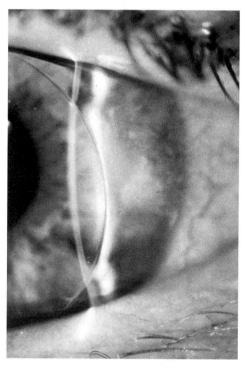

FIGURE 4-9 Gas-permeable rigid lens wearer who has developed thickening of basement membrane, neovascularization, SPK, conjunctival hyperemia, and extreme irregularity of the superficial epithelium.

prognosis for successful lens wear will be guarded and only a modified wearing schedule will be appropriate for the patient.

More recently, Korb et al have suggested reducing edge width and flattening the peripheral radius to increase the tear meniscus, thereby improving limbal wetting.[33] This would certainly be worth attempting before discontinuing lens wear. Clinically, we find that if marked limbal staining is present and cannot be eliminated, limited daily wear (at most) should be advised. When punctate staining of the limbal area occurs, we recommend discontinuing rigid lens wear. Soft lens wear can be tried, although if the patient has dry eyes, other complications related to soft lens wear are likely to develop.

Conclusion

Having reviewed the complications from RGPEW and concluded that the etiology is either metabolic or mechanical, the clinician faces the decision of whether to prescribe a medium Dk or high Dk material. The answer to this question is at least in part determined by whether the lenses are worn on an extended-wear or daily-wear basis. If the patient uses lenses only for daily wear, most materials having moderate Dk/L values 20-30 $\times 10^{-9}$ (cm $\times$ mL 0_2) /(sec $\times$ mL $\times$ mm Hg) will provide sufficient oxygen to prevent corneal hypoxia.

RGP lenses with a Dk/L of 80 $\times 10^{-9}$ (cm $\times$ mL 0_2)/(sec $\times$ mL $\times$ mm Hg) or greater will prevent hypoxia-associated complications (i.e., polymegethism, corneal edema, and microcysts) during closed-eye wear.[34] However, even with high Dk materials, mechanical problems (i.e., 3-9 o'clock SPK and lens adhesion) occur with the same incidence as with the lower Dk material.[34]

Based on this information, the clinician may question RGPEW's relative safety, especially compared to soft lens extended wear. We have compared the incidence and severity of RGPEW complications to those experienced during soft lens extended wear. In general, we find rigid lens extended wear offers an additional margin of safety over soft lens extended wear, assuming that patients with substantial lens adherence will not be allowed to continue extended wear. We also have observed a marked improvement in oxygen transmissibility of rigid materials. With newer materials being developed and approved, we believe that most metabolically related problems that occur with soft lenses will not occur with high Dk RGPEW. We also believe that the excellent tear pumping present with rigid lenses offers a substantial advantage compared to soft lenses in that trapped metabolic debris that builds up overnight is easily and quickly removed with rigid materials.

We also have studied edema recovery following sleep and found a 20% to 30% increase in the recovery rate with rigid as opposed to soft lenses. This result has been reported in the literature[35,36] and may be caused by the rapid tear flushing and exposure to high oxygen levels during open-eye periods that occur with the RGP material.

Finally, we have observed that a clean surface can be maintained on most currently available RGPEW lenses. This eliminates some of the autoimmune responses (e.g., GPC) and the red eye response associated with soft lens extended wear. Needless to say, good vision also is present most of the time with RGPEW.

In conclusion, we believe that RGP lenses offer a potential for extended wear, provided that proper follow-up care and appropriate patient instruction and management are carried out.

References

1. Klyce SD: Stromal lactate accumulation can account for corneal oedema osmotically following epithelial hypoxia in the rabbit, *J Physiol* 321:49-64, 1981.
2. Bonanno JA, Polse KA: Effect of rigid contact lens oxygen transmissibility on stromal pH in the living human eye, *Ophthalmol* 94:1350-1309, 1987.
3. Holden B, Mertz G, McNally J: Corneal swelling response to contact lenses worn under extended wear conditions, *Inv Ophthalmol Vis Sci* 24:218-226, 1983.
4. Holden B, Vannas A, Nilsson K, Efron N, Sweeney D, Kotow M, LaHood D, Guillon M: Epithelial and endothelial effects from the extended wear of contact lenses, *Curr Eye Res* 5:739, 1985.

5. Holden B, Sweeney D, Vannas A, Nilsson K, Efron N: Effects of long-term extended contact lens wear on the human cornea, *Inv Ophthalmol Vis Sci* 26:1489-1501, 1985.

6. Kenyon E, Polse K, O'Neal M: Ocular response to extended wear of hard gas-permeable lenses, *CLAO* 11:119-123, 1985.

7. MacRae S, Matsuda M, Shellans S, Rich L: The effects of hard and soft contact lenses on the corneal endothelium, *Am J Ophthalmol* 102:50-57, 1986.

8. Stocker E, Schoessler J: Corneal endothelial polymegethism induced by PMMA contact lens wear, *Inv Ophthalmol Vis Sci* 26:857-863, 1985.

9. Zantos S: Cystic formations in the corneal epithelium during extended wear of contact lenses, *ICLC* 10:128-146, 1983.

10. Polse K, Mandell R: Etiology of corneal striae accompanying hydrogel lens wear, *Invest Ophthalmol* 15:553-556, 1976.

11. Mandell R, Polse K, Fatt I: Corneal swelling caused by contact lens wear, *Arch Ophthalmol* 83:3, 1970.

12. Kenyon E, Polse K, O'Neal M: Ocular response to extended wear of hard gas-permeable lenses, *CLAO* 11(2):119-123, 1985.

13. Humphreys JA, Larke JR, Parrish ST: Microepithelial cysts observed in extended contact-lens wearing subjects, *Br J Ophthalmol* 64:888-889, 1980.

14. Polse KA, Sarver MD, Kenyon E, Bonanno JA: Gas permeable hard contact lens extended wear: ocular and visual responses to a 6-month period of wear, *CLAO* 13:31-38, 1987.

15. Kenyon E, Polse KA, Seger RG: Influence of wearing schedule on extended-wear complications, *Ophthalmol* 93:221-236, 1986.

16. Orsborn GN, Schoessler JP: Corneal endothelial polymegethism after the extended wear of rigid gas-permeable contact lenses, *Am J Optom Physiol Opt* 65:84-90, 1988.

17. Holden, B: (personal communication) *Cornea and Contact Lens Research Unit at The University of New Wales, Australia.*

18. Polse KA, Brand RJ, Cohen SR, Guillon M: Hypoxic effects on corneal morphology and function, *Inv Ophthalmol Vis Sci* 31:1542-1554, 1990.

19. Polse KA, Rivera RK, Bonnano JA: Ocular effects of hard gas-permeable-lens extended wear, *Am J Optom Physiol Opt* 65:358-364, 1988.

20. Polse KA, O'Neal MR: Oxygen requirements for extended wear, *Proceedings of the VII Congress of the European Society of Ophthalmology,* Helsinki, 269-270, 1985.

21. O'Neal M, Polse K, Sarver M: Corneal response to rigid and hydrogel lenses during eye closure, *Inv Ophthalmol Vis Sci* 25:837-841, 1984.

22. Levy B: Rigid gas-permeable lenses for extended wear—a 1-year clinical evaluation, *Am J Optom Physiol Opt* 62:889-894, 1985.

23. Schnider C, Zabkiewicz K, Terry R, et al: Unusual complications of RGP extended wear, *Am J Optom Physiol Opt(Suppl)* 63:35P, 1986.

24. Kenyon E, Polse KA, Mandell RB: Rigid contact lens adherence: incidence, severity and recovery, *Am J Optom Physiol Opt* 59:168-174, 1988.

25. Zantos SG, Zantos PO: Extended wear feasibility of gas-permeable hard lenses for myopes, *Int Eye Care* 1:66-75, 1985.

26. Lin ST, Leahy CD, Mandell RB: The effect of time, patching, and lens flexibility on RGP lens adherence, *J Am Optom Assoc* 60:182-877, 1989.

27. Kenyon E, Mandell RB, Polse KA: Lens design effects on rigid lens adherence, *J Br CL Assoc* 12:32-36, 1989.

28. Bennett BS, Egan DJ: Rigid gas-permeable lens problem solving, *J Am Optom Assoc* 57:504-511, 1986.

29. Swarbrick HA, Holden BA: Rigid gas permeable lens binding: significance and contributing factors, *Am J Optom Physiol Opt* 64:815-823, 1987.

30. Kamiya C: Cosmetic extended wear of oxygen permeable hard contact lenses: one year follow-up, *J Am Optom Assoc* 57:182-184, 1986.

31. Henry VA, Bennett ES, Forrest JF: Clinical investigation of the Paraperm EW rigid gas-permeable contact lens, *Am J Optom Physiol Opt* 64:313-320, 1987.

32. Polse KA: Changes in corneal hydration after discontinuing contact lens wear, *Am J Optom* 49(6):511-516, 1972.
33. Korb D: (personal communication) American Optometric Association Contact Lens Symposium, Boston, 1988.
34. Rivera RK, Polse KA: Corneal response to different oxygen levels during extended wear, *CLAO* 17:96-101, 1991.
35. Holden B, Sweeney D, La Hood D, Kenyon E: Corneal deswelling following overnight wear of rigid and hydrogel contact lenses, *Curr Eye Res* 7:49-53, 1988.
36. Andrasko G: Corneal deswelling response to hard and hydrogel extended wear lenses, *Inv Ophthalmol Vis Sci* 27:20, 1986.

5

Therapeutically Tinted Contact Lenses

Frank Zisman
Michael G. Harris

Key Terms

selective filtration	soft lenses	retinitis pigmentosa
X-Chrome	ultraviolet	Fuch's corneal
filters	monochromatism	dystrophy
RGP	central cone-rod	albinotic carrier
PMMA	dystrophy	syndrome

Tinted contact lenses have led to greater lens detectability, allowing an individual to find a contact lens dropped on the floor. By carefully selecting lens tint and density for selected patients, the clinician can make the floor itself more detectable.

Tints employed for the remediation of vision deficits resulting from congenital and acquired anomalies are much deeper in hue than those used for cosmesis or lens location. These lenses alter patients' color perception. However, none of the tints (including the X-Chrome lens) correct anomalous color perception.

A treatise by Zisman and Harris[1] presented regimens for remediating patient symptoms and increasing visual acuity using RGP and PMMA materials with selective wavelength transmission properties. This material will be reviewed in this chapter. Because of limited availability, high cost, and poor uniformity among lenses of the same material, soft lenses tinted with therapeutic dyes were not recommended at that time.

Soft contact lens therapeutic tints have since become a viable option. The most common and readily available tint is the X-Chrome type or magenta tint, which is useful for patients suffering from cone-rod dystrophies and bright-to-dark mobility problems, and with some incipient cataract patients. Optical Designs, Adventures in Color, and Kontur Contact Lens supplied the tinted products cited in this presentation. The two former companies tint provided lenses, and the latter supplies lenses tinted on their own base material (a medium water content lens). Presently, the only company to offer ultraviolet-blocking tints is CooperVision. This type of selective cut-off filter should be a property of all contact lens materials.

The X-Chrome and Color Vision

The introduction of the X-Chrome contact lens in the late 1950s was supposed to bring an end to one of nature's mistakes—anomalous color perception. Presumptions about anomalous color perception and the X-Chrome lens' ability to correct it have proven incorrect. However, the lens has been proven a useful tool for other vision anomalies that will be discussed later.

Individuals who had failed pseudoisochromatic color (PIC) plate tests could often properly identify plates while wearing the tinted lens on one eye and viewing the test with both eyes. Proper identification of the figures on the plates was interpreted as restoration of normal color vision. Patients with normal color perception viewing the plates through the device see some of the plates rendered more dramatically. A clue often missed by these normal subjects was that other figures became less apparent. The magenta lens transmitted the blues and reds reflected from the PIC plates and darkened the greens.

The controverted explanation was, "... red deficient by nature in one eye, and induced green deficient in the other—both eyes open—the patient would be normal by default. In fact, the design of the PIC test has been circumvented.

The intent of PIC tests is to place a symbol of given hue and chroma on a background of hues and chromas that fall on a line in color space that can be confused as being the same by patients with color deficiencies. Saturation of the chromas can be varied to help define the depth or degree of color deficiency. Each plate in the series tests along a specific color confusion axis. The figure's reflected brightness and the background for all chromas are held equal so that brightness will not clue the observer. To ensure this, the tests are designed to be administered under specific lighting conditions such as C.I.E. illuminant "C" (designed to represent late-morning, northern spring daylight). Some tests have been designed to be administered under illuminant "A," or a 100-watt tungsten bulb.

Lighting conditions have a minimal effect on patients with normal color perception except in the extreme. Illumination can affect testing results for some patients with color perception deficiencies.

A surface's perceived color is the result of light reflected from the pigments in that surface. A red surface reflects red wavelengths from the illuminant and absorbs all other wavelengths. If a red figure were placed upon a black surface of equal reflection and the entire area illuminated with a mercury vapor lamp, no figure would be observed, even by a patient with normal color perception. Mercury vapor lamps emit no red light, so none is available to be reflected. The black background absorbs all wavelengths of light, and the red figure absorbs all wavelengths except red. Because no red is present to reflect, the figure merges into the background.

A red-blind individual does not have photoreceptors to detect red light. Under the same scenario, but using normal daylight, a red figure on a black background would remain submerged because no photoreceptors are present to detect reflected red light. This oversimplification can be used to illustrate how filters and lighting alter perception.

As we have seen, the illuminant can affect the wavelengths of light available to be reflected. Biasing the light toward red by using a common tungsten household lamp provides more red to be reflected by red-reflecting pigments, and less blue to be absorbed by blue-absorbing pigments. A relative brightness gradient is established across the PIC plate, and a patient with a red color deficiency is able to detect a "brighter" pattern on an otherwise color-confusing background. Detection is not based upon hue or chroma, but by brightness differences.

An alternative method of affecting a brightness gradient is to place a selective cut-off filter between the observer and the object. Here we use a red filter that transmits only red light. Red objects observed through this filter appear brighter than other colored objects, which are darkened. Even a patient with protanopia will see the relative brightness difference. This is not a color vision function, but rather a brightness discrimination function, reliant upon a different set of nerve pathways.

The ability to pass a PIC test with an X-Chrome lens has been misinterpreted as color vision normalization. In his doctoral thesis, Labissioner[2] demonstrated a shift in hue discrimination in patients with color deficiencies away from their primary color deficiency toward an alternative color deficiency. Unilaterally, patients with protanopia displayed deuteranopia. Binocularly, hue discrimination remained poor. The argument, ". . . protan one eye, deutan the other, and normal by default binocularly," did not prove true.

Testing with the Farnsworth D-15 dichotomous test demonstrates the same results. Color confusions are still made by X-Chrome type lens wearers. Normal results are not achieved.

An issue not dealt with in the literature promoting these filters is the Pulfricht effect—simple and chromatic. The filtering of only one eye causes a shift in binocular spatial perception. A demonstration of this effect can be observed in patients with both normal and deficient color perception by placing a red filter in front of one eye while the individual observes a pendulum. Without the filter, the pendulum traverses a predicted physical space (i.e., back and forth in a straight line). With the filter, the pendulum appears to swing in an arc, with the direction of the arc determined by the eye filtered.

Adaptation to the Pulfricht effect has not been demonstrated with individuals wearing this device or with those who wear a neutral-density filter in the other eye (although less noticeable, a color-specific component can be observed). Spatial disruptions while driving or walking in traffic should be a cause for concern, at least in the early stages of use of this type of device.

Once the nature of the change in perception is understood by practitioner and patient, definite indications exist for use of this therapy with selected patients with color deficiencies. One example is the 55-year-old protanomalous handyman who has used a gauged meter when attending to electrical repairs, but has had to replace the now-defective device with current technology—a red–light-emitting diode (LED) display meter. If the device cannot be exchanged for one with a different color display, a selective cut-off filter would make the LEDs appear brighter. A filter will prove more cost effective than a job retraining program.

Individuals with color deficiencies trying to use a color–vision-altering device to obtain a job requiring color-normal vision should be viewed with suspicion. The police department in Fremont, California, recanted on allowing the use of X-Chrome type lenses, because once on the force officers did not wear the devices. Reasons given for discontinuation included poor comfort, distorted vision, and comments from the public about the fitted eye's unusual appearance.*

These devices can be helpful for individuals with color deficiencies who have to differentiate between limited and specific colors, such as a diver who has to tell the difference between a red and green nozzle to hook up an undersea gas line. They are less worthwhile if a large number of color variants must be dealt with or if color rendering or naming is involved. The lenses have applications other than for assistance in color differentiation. Healthful fitting of these devices presents an added challenge to the prescriber.

---

*Personal communication, Police Chief, Fremont, California, 1980.

Fitting Procedures

Soft Contact Lenses

The development of soft lens disinfection systems that do not employ hydrogen peroxide (which tends to bleach tints over time) has helped make therapeutically tinted soft lenses a viable option. These lens materials can be accurately reproduced for hue and chroma across each lens and among lenses. They do not fade appreciably over their expected lives when the newer disinfection systems are used with them. The simplified hygiene regimens also work better for patients with the conditions presented in this chapter.

Fitting therapeutically tinted soft lenses is no different than fitting standard soft lenses. The practitioner can fit the standard lens of choice and send that lens to a lab for tinting, or (if the tint is lab proprietary) fit a clear trial lens and then order a similarly tinted lens. Therapeutic tinting does not appear to alter the fitting characteristics of spherical low water content soft lenses. Changes in oxygen permeability with soft lens tinting have not been officially reported in the literature. However, an in-house study performed by Ocu-Ease on its 53% and 65% water materials (ocufilcon B) using Fatt's method of determining Dk showed an approximate 15% increase in oxygen transmission through each lens material, comparing clear to cosmetically tinted. Therapeutic tint densities were not tested. Also using Fatt's method, Pilkington Barnes Hind technicians studied changes in their materials' Dk with visibility tints. They claimed no change for the CSI materials (crofilcon A), but noted a possible 1% to 5% increase in Dk for bifilcon A materials.*

CLINICAL PEARL

Therapeutic tinting does not appear to alter the fitting characteristics of spherical low water content soft lenses.

Medium water content lenses appear to steepen slightly and shrink approximately 0.2 mm in diameter with cosmetic tinting. This was not noted with visibility tinting. This does not substantially alter the fitting characteristics of spherical lenses, but in marginal fitting performance a flatter base curve might be considered. Medium water content torics (specifically Ocu-Ease and Hydrocurve III) need a flatter base curve after therapeutic tinting to retain maximal lens position and orientation. This is not necessary with Ciba Vision's Torisoft low

---

*Both in-house studies were related as personal communications to the authors.

water toric lenses. Tinted Torisoft lenses performed in the same manner when they were trial fitted as clear lenses.

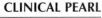

CLINICAL PEARL

Medium water content lenses appear to steepen slightly and shrink approximately 0.2 mm in diameter with cosmetic tinting. This was not noted with visibility tinting.

The red or X-Chrome type tint is the most readily available therapeutic tint for soft lenses. The spectral transmissions for this tint in three densities are presented in Figure 5-1. Red 3 by Optical Designs and X-Chrome type by Kontur Contact Lens have spectral transmissions that superimpose when the lens material is tinted. Transmissions through these tints are a good approximation to the Alberta II Ruby-red, gas-permeable lens or the X-Chrome PMMA lens. This tint has proven useful in treating cone-rod dystrophic vision and severe photophobia.

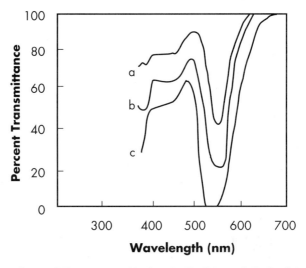

FIGURE 5-1 Optical Designs **A,** Red 1; **B,** Red 2; and **C,** Red 3. Red 3 and Kontur X-Chrome type tint superimpose. Transmission characteristics of these tints are almost identical except for density, suggesting either dilutions of the same dye or different time exposures of a given dye. Base lens material does not appear to affect transmission characteristics. Red 3 was on a low water CibaSoft lens and the Kontur dye was on Kontur's medium water lens. Superimposition of the two curves suggests the same dye.

Red 1 and 2 tints from Optical Designs have the same transmission characteristics of the Red 3 tint, but with less density. These tints are useful in managing milder asthenopias related to brightness and glare, improving visual resolution in incipient cataract, and lessening patient difficulties related to rod-cone dystrophy and sudden bright-to-dim luminance changes (such as entering a building from a bright environment).

Patients wearing these tints report a shift in the environment's perceived color. These lenses transmit minimally in the blue (400 nm to 480 nm) and not at all in the middle of the visual spectrum. They are better tolerated psychologically by wearers than those that do not transmit in the blue.

Some custom tinting labs will render a "dense" version of any of their standard colors upon request. Reproducibility for these subjectively requested tints is questionable. For cosmetic reasons (as will be discussed later when dealing with rigid materials) it might be desirable to use one or more of these "dense" versions.

Rigid Contact Lenses

Precise fitting of some of the new rigid gas-permeable (RGP) and therapeutically tinted contact lenses can pose a problem for the traditional trial lens fitter. One property of these materials, although beneficial to the patient, limits the usefulness of fluorescein as a fitting aid. The inherent ultraviolet (UV) and short wavelength blocking and absorbing characteristics of these materials afford safer and better vision, but do not readily transmit visible light in the region needed to use fluorescein. This may be caused by silicon absorbency and reflection, material additives, or both. Davis and Bennett[3] have suggested methods of enhancing fluorescein's usefulness through the use of selective "exciter" filters.

CLINICAL PEARL

The inherent ultraviolet (UV) and short wavelength blocking and absorbing characteristics of these materials afford safer and better vision, but do not readily transmit visible light in the region needed to use fluorescein.

Clear lenses can be considered tinted if by prescription they are designed to eliminate part of the visual spectrum, including the zone that contains UV. A lens made from a material that reduces spectral transmittance is a tinted lens.

Therapeutically or deeply tinted contact lenses are most often prescribed to individuals with reduced visual acuity. RGP tints, when available, are superior to soft or polymethylmethacrylate (PMMA) lenses. The major drawback of PMMA material is its lack of oxygen transmissibility. Presently, durability is the major disadvantage of soft materials.

In the past, PMMA wearers with marginal metabolic and physical lens fits have had their problems resolved by being moved into RGP materials, often without lens redesign. Because the RGP materials tend to be light, they either moved more (thus enhancing tear pumping) or fit higher under the superior lid, facilitating lens movement and tear flushing. Both enhance corneal health. More recently, RGP lenses have been designed to fit superiorly on the cornea or slightly under the lids to facilitate greater corneal oxygenation. PMMA lenses relied upon flat, corneal compressive fits to obtain these actions, which often left the patients with corneal edema during wear and after removal, and spectacle blur for hours after lens removal. Compressive fits and edema led to corneal erosion and lens intolerance.

Fitting therapeutically tinted PMMA and RGP materials requires care in maintaining corneal alignment with minimal apical clearance and full pupil coverage, even after blinks. To obtain full pupil coverage, slightly larger lens diameters might be required than those usually fit. We recommend using tricurve rather than bicurve back surface lens designs. If aspherics are employed, a slightly increased "Q" (0.03 mm to 0.05 mm) factor for 9.0 mm to 10.0 mm lenses should be applied to keep the lenses central on the cornea, after achieving what would otherwise be a best fit for a nontinted lens. Care should be taken to avoid excessive central pooling or intermediate bearing.

Initial fitting should be done with clear lenses in the material to be prescribed, so that fluorescein patterns can be observed. After an ideal fit is determined, the tint type and density can be determined with a modified parameter tint set. To obtain the desired filter density or spectral transmission, lens thicknesses of 0.17 mm to 0.20 mm are required. Lens flexure in most materials available today is negligible in these thicknesses. This should be taken into consideration during the initial clear lens fitting. An ideal 0.12 mm center thickness trial fit may not center in a 0.20 mm center thickness final fit, because the final lens' mass will be greater.

After an ideal fit is attained, follow-up examinations should be performed at regular intervals of no more than 6 months. Lens performance should be assessed for movement, centration, comfort, and clarity. Fluorescein patterns should be assessed and special attention paid to residual fluorescein marking of the ocular tissues when the lenses are removed. Because these lenses are fit thicker than standard RGP lenses for most patients with myopia, oxygen transmittance is reduced, and central corneal clouding (CCC) must be looked for upon lens removal. Grade 2 or greater clouding necessitates a fitting readjustment. For PMMA fits where Dk = 0, CCC remains the problem it has been in the past. It should be assumed that grade 1 is baseline and always present. Reduced or modified wear schedules should be employed for patients needing PMMA-based tinted lenses.

Material Availability

The availability of therapeutic tints in rigid materials is limited to the X-Chrome, the Alberta II red lens in RGP, and to blue, green, amber, brown, red, and gray lenses in PMMA. Glasflex manufactures PMMA materials in buttons that can be lathed. It was the original manufacturer of X-Chrome lens materials.

The X-Chrome and Glasflex Ruby-Red 2241-1 lenses are actually magenta—blue is transmitted with the red. The spectral properties of the Alberta II red lens closely approximate those of the X-Chrome, with 5% greater transmission in the blue. The "leakage" of blue through these lenses is most likely why they were initially successful with patients with color deficiencies. Red-only transmitting lenses are often rejected.

Tints can be interchanged for some ocular conditions, if the cosmesis of the preferred lens is unacceptable. Trial fitting with various tints will facilitate final lens selection. A reduced fitting set of tinted lenses with base curves of 8.13 mm, 7.76 mm, and 7.42 mm in a 9.2 mm diameter, modified-contour configuration should suffice.

Reasons for Fitting Therapeutically Tinted Contact Lenses

Clinical experience with patients with monochromatism and other retinal conditions indicates that better vision performance and comfort occur with contact lens correction compared to a similar tint in a spectacle format. Full pupillary coverage that limits peripheral glare, and greater selective spectral transmission because of the reduced number of optical surfaces are reasons for improved performance. Spectacle tints allow light to enter the pupil from above, from below, and from the sides of the glasses. Rear surface reflections also reduce vision quality. Side shields and hat brims employed to reduce glare also reduce patient mobility.

CLINICAL PEARL

Full pupillary coverage that limits peripheral glare, and greater selective spectral transmission because of the reduced number of optical surfaces are reasons for improved performance.

Ocular Conditions and Appropriate Tints

A number of conditions can benefit from therapeutically tinted contact lenses. These include the following conditions:
1. Monochromatism
2. Central cone-rod dystrophy
3. Retinitis pigmentosa
4. Incipient cataract
5. Fuch's corneal dystrophy
6. Albinotic carrier syndrome

Monochromatism

Patients with rod monochromatism possess only rods in their retinas. Light above mesopic levels causes extreme discomfort for these individuals. Although visual acuity and resolution will remain poor, vision comfort and patient mobility can be greatly enhanced by lenses that bring ambient retinal illumination to mesopic or lower levels. Useful lenses for these patients are The Dark Gray 6077 and Dark Brown 2285 lenses by Glasflex, and the Alberta II lens (Figure 5-2). These lenses reduce retinal illumination to less than 20% where the rods are most sensitive (i.e., approximately 510 nm), placing them in a comfortable mesopic range.

Patients with cone monochromatism generally have some rod vision. Although these patients have severely reduced visual acuity, some enhancement may occur with proper tint selection, depending on the type of cone monochromatism. Because of the parsity of blue cones,

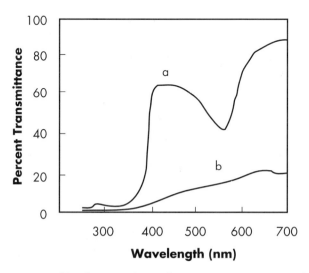

FIGURE 5-2 A, Glasflex Dark Pink 2241-5, 0.18 mm thickness; **B,** Glasflex Dark Gray 6077, 0.20 mm thickness.

patients with blue cone monochromatism will notice no substantial acuity improvement. Those with red or green cone monochromatism may obtain incremental benefits in resolution.

The lens of choice for patients with blue cone monochromatism is the Glasflex Dark Blue 1077-2 (Figure 5-3), with a maximum transmittance of 80% at 440 nm falling to approximately 45% by 510 nm (Figure 5-4). For both red and green cone monochromatism, the Glasflex Ruby-Red 2241-1, X-Chrome, and Alberta II red lenses have been the lenses of choice. Patients with green cone monochromatism also may benefit from the Glasflex Dark Green 2240-1 filter if the Alberta lens' cosmesis is a problem (Figure 5-5).

The rationale for fitting patients with monochromatism with selective cut-off filters is straightforward: bias retinal illumination toward the available photoreceptors and bring overall retinal illumination to mesopic levels for patient comfort. This rationale can be applied to patients suffering from retinal dystrophies.

Electrophysiological evidence exists for shared rod-cone pathways in primate retina.[4] Cone signals appear to inhibit rod signals as light levels increase. Leeper and Copenhagen[5] showed selective anatomical connections between rods and red type cones in turtle retina via horizontal cells. Coletta and Adams[6] demonstrated in humans that laterally mediated steady-state signals from rods alter foveal sensitivity for cone flicker detection and that a special relationship exists between red cones and rods. However, they tested only for the red cone condition. This observation in humans is supported by Heis and Mullen[7] and Frumkee et al.[8]

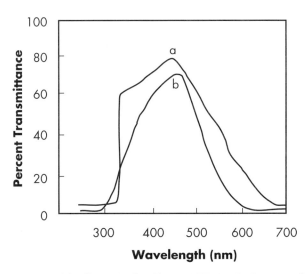

FIGURE 5-3 A, Glasflex Dark Blue 1077-2, 0.12 mm thickness; **B,** Glasflex Blue 1077, 0.20 mm thickness.

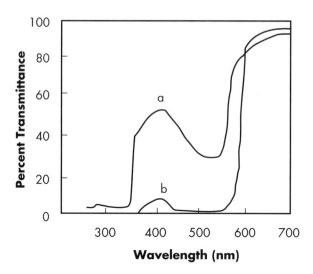

FIGURE 5-4 **A,** Glasflex Ruby Red 2241-1 and X-Chrome, 0.12 mm thickness; **B,** Alberta II red, 0.20 mm thickness. Note how center thickness affects the relative transmission, especially in the blue end of the spectrum.

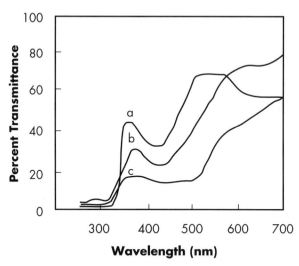

FIGURE 5-5 **A,** Glasflex Dark Green 2240-1, 0.20 mm thickness; **B,** Glasflex Medium Brown 2285-2, 0.20 mm thickness; **C,** Glasflex Dark Brown 2285, 0.19 mm thickness.

Although evidence points to red cone-rod-shared pathways, opponent color theory (intercone interaction) would lead to strong speculation that green cones also share rod pathways. Clinically, patients with protanopia and deuteranopia do not have different rod-related vision problems. The experience of Zisman and Adams[9] with a patient with green-cone monochromatism and his selective filter choices supports this assumption.

Central Cone-Rod Dystrophy

Central cone-rod dystrophy is a disorder of macular vision that produces reduced visual acuity, acquired color vision deficiency, mild retinal arterial narrowing, macular pigmentary changes, reduced cone electroretinogram, reduced cone dark adaptation, and central scotomas.[10] Color vision can become scotopic, and visual acuity falls to between 20/200 and 20/400.

Zisman and Harris[11] established a methodology to determine cut-off filter selection and to determine how the filter was increasing visual acuity for a patient with central cone-rod dystrophy. Using the evidence and arguments presented previously, Glasflex Ruby-Red 2241-1 and Alberta II red RGP lenses were employed, significantly improving visual acuity from 20/240 to 20/50 and providing good visual comfort.

We postulated that cone-rod dystrophy reduces rod inhibition, allowing both rod and weak cone signals down shared pathways, with rod signals predominating and causing "visual noise" during photopic conditions. This noise was described as "glare" by the patient, but was different from the "glare" he had experienced when his visual system was normal (i.e., from surfaces and side lighting, and the scattering he noticed when his spectacles were dusty or oily).

Although the resultant visual acuity was identical to that occurring with the Ruby-Red and Alberta II lenses, the patient favored the Alberta II lenses because of their slightly greater blue transmission (10% compared to 5% for the PMMA lenses). This slight increase in blue transmission allowed him to see the sky as blue. With the Glasflex Ruby-Red lenses, the sky appeared red.

Retinitis Pigmentosa

Retinitis pigmentosa (RP) is essentially a rod-cone dystrophy, the opposite of central cone-rod dystrophy. RP is predominantly inherited, via numerous modes, and also can be found in conjunction with trisomy 21 (Down syndrome) and as a result of rubella during pregnancy. RP can only be fully diagnosed after electroretinography, because many other conditions can present an ocular fundus picture similar to retinitis pigmentosa. Among these are commotio retinae, syphilis, and ocular phlebitis, all of which are less specific in their modes of effecting retinal desensitization.

Night vision and peripheral vision problems are the first to manifest in a patient with RP. Central vision problems ensue, including reduced central visual acuity and acquired color vision deficiency. Although it is usual to observe vitreoretinal interface and posterior polar lenticular changes (both of which contribute to reduced central acuity), the acquired color vision deficiency measurable within the first 7 years of onset points to central nerve pathway disruption.

Selective cut-off filters can reduce the abberant input from a degenerating rod system and can enhance the quality if not quantity of central vision. Zisman and Harris[11] used RGP cut-off filter contact lenses with one RP patient. The patient's visual acuity was 20/200 in each eye and her visual field was 10 degrees in subtense. This patient kept high levels of incandescent lighting in her home, but could not tolerate bright outdoor or fluorescent lighting. She had selected a pair of deeply rose-tinted commercial sunglasses for use outdoors and while shopping.

Using Alberta II red lenses, this patient was able to obtain 20/80 visual acuity in each eye, sufficient to read a newspaper with a 2× magnifier at a comfortable distance. She also was able to tolerate supermarket lighting and move comfortably from bright outdoor lighting into her house with less "theater effect" than with the sunglasses. Once indoors, she was able to remove her lenses.

Because of the inherent red shift with incandescent bulbs, much less sub-500 nm light was present in her home, causing less rod stimulation than under the other conditions. Her contact lenses therefore simply reduced her indoor retinal illumination by 20%. She now wears her contact lenses only when going outdoors, which she does more frequently than before contact lens filters were fitted to her. She claims her vision is sharper and more comfortable. Lens handling is not a problem, because the deep tint permits easy location and the rigid construction permits easy manipulation.

Incipient Cataract and Corneal Glare Sources

During the early to middle stages of cataractogenesis and in the middle to early late stages of Fuch's corneal dystrophy, glare secondary to light scattering in the ocular media can cause discomfort and incremental losses in visual acuity. Reports concerning the Corning CPF series filters have indicated that the apparent visibility of the environment can be enhanced for patients suffering from these symptoms. CPF 511 and 527 spectacle cut-off filters appear to be of greatest help to this group. When using these tints, residual back surface lens reflections and glare from light entering the eye from above and from the sides of the lenses are reduced with side shields and hat brims.

This patient group's mobility can be enhanced using contact lens cut-off filters. Full pupillary coverage by the tinted lens prevents stray light from entering the eye, eliminating the need for side shields and hat brims. CPF tints can best be approximated by the Alberta II red lens and similar tints in PMMA and soft gel lenses. Trial fitting with these tints should be performed to determine ideal density and color. Glasflex Medium Brown 2285-2 or Dark Brown 2285 also may be appropriate for some patients. The cosmesis of these two latter tints might prove more acceptable to patients with naturally blue or light-colored irides. It has been our experience that fair-complected

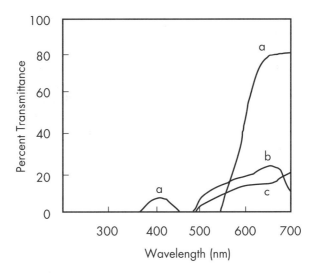

FIGURE 5-6 **A,** Corning Medical Optics CPF 550 darkened transmittance; **B,** Vuarnet spectacle transmittance; **C,** Bolle IREX 100 spectacle transmittance.

individuals have often opted for the brown lenses for cosmetic reasons. These lenses give the wearer a visual perception of the world much like that noted by wearers of Bolle IREX 100 spectacle tints (Figure 5-6).

To obtain the desired transmissions from the red lenses it will be necessary to reduce the center thicknesses of the lenses to approximately 0.10 mm (approximating the CPF 527). Contact lens flexure may pose a problem. If flexure is a problem, the Medium Brown 2285-2 and Dark Pink 2241-5 lenses by Glasflex may be employed. More than one of the tints might perform with the same suitability in terms of vision quality, but patients might have a preference as to how they would like to see the world or how they would like the world to see them. For these reasons, trial tint fitting is most helpful and will influence this therapy's long-term success.

Albinotic Carrier Syndrome

Albinism and ocular albinism are well-documented genetic conditions. Among the very fair complected, there exists a subpopulation who are not albinotic or ocularly albinotic, but carry recessive genetic traits for this condition. A careful history will show that as very young children these individuals had pale blue irides and almost translucent hair. As they aged, their hair and irides darkened, similar to the darkening that occurs with tyrosine-positive albinotics.

These patients present with symptoms of extreme photophobia. Although their vision is correctable to 20/20, when refractive error is present refraction must take place in a dim room with a reduced illumination chart. Pupillary dilation does not generally cause a minus shift in the resultant power, because the patients' extreme photosensitivity leaves them with a relatively normal pupil size in the dim illumination.

These individuals often display volitional or behavioral nystagmus that can be controlled to minimize discomfort and accommodative insufficiency secondary to avoiding near tasks. They or their families may volunteer that their home environment is a "dark cave."

These patients are often listed as visually disabled because of the severity of their photophobia. They are excellent candidates for selective cut-off filters.

Corning CPF filters have proven helpful for this patient group. At the Vision Functions Clinic of the University of California School of Optometry, patients reported good vision comfort in areas that were uncomfortable without these spectacle lenses. However, when given the lenses on a trial basis, the majority of patients opted not to wear them regularly because the cosmesis was unacceptable. Many tired of repeated unsolicited comments about the unusual appearance of their glasses and all were bothered by peripheral glare from around and behind the lenses.

Less obvious and more effective, the Alberta II red lenses proved helpful for a patient fitted by Zisman, Zisman, and Harris.[12] These lenses provided excellent vision comfort indoors while allowing adequate indoor illumination for the patient's family to move about the house. They also were acceptable to the patient at dawn and dusk outdoors. A deep rose plus gray 80% tinted pair of sunglasses was prescribed (with distance prescription) for use outdoors during the day. The patient found accommodation through her full-distance myopic correction uncomfortable. Given her proximity to presbyopia, vision training would not have been worthwhile. Indoors, her mild myopic refractive error did not pose a problem. Contact lens power in each lens was +0.25, effectively giving her a +2.00 add. She finds this ideal because she is learning word processing, an impossible task when she was on vision disability.

Although the patient was fair complected, the cosmesis of the deep red lenses was well accepted. Unsolicited comments from family and friends were abundant but not wholly negative, and the vision comfort afforded by the lenses outweighed the initial attention garnered because of them.

Initial fitting of the patient proved challenging. Nystagmoid movements and narrowing apertures during keratometry made taking K readings less than routine. After initial trial lenses were selected for fitting, fluorescein assessment with the cobalt filter proved uncomfortable for the patient. However, after the final filtered lenses were prescribed, adaptation was rapid. Clear lenses were used for fitting, and are used to assess cornea/contact lens relationships during follow-up assessments. Clear-lens evaluations are still uncomfortable for the patient. A modified procedure has been adopted using fluorescein only to assess staining after lens dynamics are judged. Lens performance assessment with white light while the patient wears her filtered lenses does not appear uncomfortable.

Conclusion

Therapeutically tinted contact lenses can provide a useful means of remediating symptomatic and functional visual anomalies in individuals with congenital and acquired visual deficiencies. The healthful fitting of these materials requires technical foresight and careful methodology. The clinician must consider the whole patient rather than just the disorder to facilitate successful, long-term remediation of the problem. Individuals with perceptual problems are acutely sensitive to solutions that generate new problems.

Useful and cost-effective materials are available in PMMA, RGP, and hydrogel lens designs. Because of the limited tint selection in commonly used present day materials, the practitioner may have to review the "ancient literature" to appropriately prescribe PMMA-based tints.

A blond individual with early cataractogenic contrast loss may opt for slightly less distinct vision and a more normal appearance. Without the option of alternative tints, a successful tool may end up in the bathroom drawer. The drawer will see no better.

As with low vision aids, therapeutically tinted contact lenses must be prescribed for specific conditions. Specific vision conditions are more easily remedied than diffuse or global conditions.

The devices must be methodically tried on. Normal observers' perceptions through tints are difficult to correlate scientifically to actual performance. Patton et al[13] demonstrated in patients with normal color perception that selective filters at threshold performed predictably regardless of tint and subjective evaluation. "High contrast" tints caused the same decreases in vision performance as "general" tints, based upon tint density and the targets viewed. Studies on CPF lenses for patients with normal color perception have been inconclusive at best. They have based their results in part on regimens employing assessment-utilizing black on white targets.

Proper selection of cut-off filters for individuals with specific perception disorders can remediate symptoms, and in some instances enhance visual acuity. When applied in a contact lens regimen, these filters can provide greater visual benefits than when applied in spectacle lenses.

References

1. Zisman F, Harris MG: The uses of therapeutically tinted contact lenses for vision disorders, *Probl in Optom* Vol 2, no. 4, 704-714, 1990.
2. Labissioner P (ed): "The X-Chrome lens," *Int Cont Lens Clin* I/4:55-88, 1974; and Doctoral Thesis, University of California School of Optometry, 1973.
3. Davis LJ, Bennett ES: Fluorescein patterns in UV-absorbing rigid contact lenses, *Spectrum* 4(8) Aug:49-54, 1989.
4. Gouras P, Link K: Rod and cone interaction in dark adapted monkey ganglion cells, *J Physiol* 184:499-510, 1966.
5. Leeper HF, Copenhagen DR: Mixed rod-cone responses in horizontal cells of snapping turtle retina, *Vis Res* 19:407-412, 1979.
6. Coletta NJ, Adams AJ: Rod-cone interaction in flicker detection, *Vis Res* 24: 1333-1340, 1984.
7. Heis RF, Mullen KT: Supression of the central cone signal under mesopic conditions, *ARVO Abstr* 1:16, 1982.
8. Frumkee TE, Egsteinsson T, Arden GB: Tonic inhibition of red-cone pathways by dark adapted rods, *ARVO Abstr* 84:114, 1985.
9. Zisman F, Adams AJ: A green-cone monochromat, case report, grand rounds, University of California, Berkeley, California, 1983.
10. Krill, AE: Hereditary retinal and choroidal diseases: *Clinical Characteristics*, 1977, Harper and Row, Vol 2, pp. 8-25 and 466-467.
11. Zisman F, Harris MG: Filter enhanced visual acuity in a case of central cone-rod dystrophy, *Color Vis Defic IX* 189-194, 1989.
12. Zisman F, Zisman KR, Harris MG: Transmissions and utility of therapeutically tinted contact lenses, *Color Vis Defic X* 251-256, 1991.
13. Patton GA, Rhone JE, Shoji NE: Ophthalmic tints for hunters and marksmen: effects on visual performance, Doctoral Thesis, University of California School of Optometry, Berkeley, California, 1982.

Acknowledgments

The authors would like to thank Cynthia Bancer, Glasflex Corp., Quido A Cappelli Ophthalmics, Richard J Kirmil, PROCON, Chuck Vermette, OcuEase, Carl J Moore, Concise Contact Lens, Kontur Contact Lens, Optical Designs, Adventures in Color, and Dr. Joseph Bonnano for technical and physical support.

6

Visual Problems with Contact Lenses

Noel A. Brennan
Nathan Efron

Key Terms

contact lens	refractive error	corneal shape
soft lens	anterior ocular	binocular vision
vision loss	tissues	
contrast sensitivity function		

Contact lenses are fitted to correct vision defects. It is therefore paradoxical that of all the topics discussed in contact lens literature, vision correction receives so little attention. The causes of vision loss during contact lens wear are not always obvious, and a definitive diagnosis may be difficult because of the transient or inconsistent nature of the problem.

Many factors may lead to vision problems during daily wear of hydrogel lenses. This chapter will review the causes and mechanisms of these conditions, and present management plans for maintaining patient satisfaction.

This chapter has been reproduced from Efron N, Brennan NA: How to manage complaints of vision loss during contact lens wear. (Ch. 2). In *The International Contact Lens Year Book*, London, 1994, Saunders.

Measurement of Vision

General Description of Vision Loss

Decreased vision performance during contact lens wear may present in many forms. The nature of vision loss is a key factor in determining the basis of the symptom. The following list provides a summary of characteristics that can be used to describe vision loss:

- Severity (marked or severe)
- Consistency (constant or fluctuating)
- Onset (immediate or delayed)
- Distance or near
- Persistence during lens wear
- Persistence following lens removal
- Haze
- Glare

Contrast Sensitivity Function

Patients frequently report problems with vision performance during contact lens wear, despite good acuity as measured using standard high-contrast test charts. To explain the basis for these complaints, more sophisticated assessment of vision status through measurement of contrast sensitivity has been applied. The results of these studies have been equivocal. Some experiments have found significant losses in vision performance during lens wear[1, 2]; others have found no loss[3, 4] or even improvement in vision performance.[5] Many variables should be considered when assessing the results of these studies, including lens fit, water content, duration of wear, adaptation of the subject to lens wear, the experience of the experimental subjects in making judgments of sensitivity, and the experimental protocol used.

When the results of these studies are considered, contact lenses appear to provide vision performance comparable to spectacles. Nonetheless, several noteworthy findings have arisen from contrast sensitivity experiments.[4] Grey[2] reported that contrast sensitivity losses may be present during adaptation to lens wear, although Nowozyckyj et al.[4] were unable to confirm this finding. Certainly, any vision decrement that occurs during adaptation resolves with time to the extent that vision may be slightly superior with contact lens wear in the adapted subject.[4]

High- and Low-Contrast Acuity Charts

Measurement of the contrast sensitivity function is the most thorough psychophysical method to assess vision; however, such electronic laboratory-based techniques are time consuming and expensive. For the clinical setting, simpler and more practical methods of assessing vision are required.

Contrast sensitivity in patients without major pathology can be described by determining two points on the function: the maximum frequency that can be resolved (that is, the best acuity) and the maximum sensitivity in the low-contrast range.[6] High- and low-contrast charts based on the logMAR scale (logMAR is an anagram for logarithm of the minimum angle of resolution[7]) enable these points to be determined (Figure 6-1). Failure to achieve acuity comparable to spectacles for the high-contrast charts means a refractive problem is likely; procedures for identifying an uncorrected refractive state should be instituted. Failure to achieve optimal results for the low-contrast chart, in combination with normal high-contrast acuity, indicates that factors other than refractive state, such as lens fit, epithelial edema, or lens deposition should be investigated.

Glare Source

Certain lens-induced ocular abnormalities such as epithelial edema increase light scattering. Consequently, vision is degraded in the presence of a glare source. Glare sensitivity is best detected using a simple light source in combination with low-contrast acuity charts.[8] One of the more useful applications of such a procedure is in the differentiation of epithelial and stromal edema.[8] Despite its potential advantages, glare testing has yet to be fully exploited in the clinical setting.

General Strategies for Investigating Vision Loss

An important consideration in investigating vision loss during contact lens wear is whether the loss can be ascribed to the lens or some underlying ocular abnormality. One strategy is to determine visual

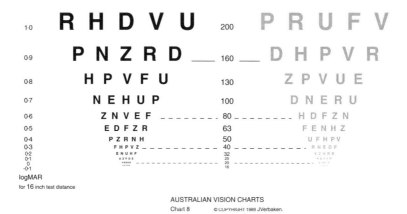

AUSTRALIAN VISION CHARTS
Chart 8   © COPYRIGHT 1989 JVerbaken.

FIGURE 6-1 High (90%) and low (10%) contrast logMAR charts designed for testing vision at near distance. (Courtesy of Jos Verbaken, Australian Vision Charts).

acuity after lens removal. Restoration of normal vision upon lens removal suggests that the problem is lens based, whereas prolonged vision loss points toward an ocular basis for the symptoms.

CLINICAL PEARL

Restoration of normal vision upon lens removal suggests that the problem is lens based, whereas prolonged vision loss points toward an ocular basis for the symptoms.

Whether the visual loss occurs in one or both eyes can provide additional clues as to the source of the problem. Unilateral vision reduction is likely to be lens related or caused by isolated pathological conditions, whereas bilateral vision loss may be caused by more general pathology, such as toxicity and allergic conditions.

Researchers have postulated that in addition to the optically degrading effect of defocus, the cornea/contact lens system may produce aberrations that cause a reduction in that component of the optical signal that provides medium- or low-frequency visual information. Consequently, the contrast sensitivity function of the patient would be expected to decrease.

Residual Uncorrected Refractive Error

In assessing vision loss during contact lens wear, the first factor to consider is whether the loss is caused by inappropriate refractive correction.

Spherical Error

An obvious cause of major vision loss is lens displacement or loss. Soft lenses are generally so comfortable that patients may be unaware of them during normal wear; it follows that a patient can be unaware of lens displacement or loss.

Shifts in the refractive error of the eye can account for vision loss. Alternately, lens power may have been ordered incorrectly in the first place or supplied incorrectly by the laboratory. When confronted with refractive inconsistencies, the practitioner must be prepared to conduct a full refractive workup and accurately measure the power of the lens.

Flexure of a soft lens over the cornea can result in power changes because of the entrapment of tear films of various thickness beneath the lens. Weissman's[9] general model predicts that low minus thin lenses entrap tear layers of low volume and minimum power, whereas low plus lenses can entrap tear layers of greater volume and significant power (up to −2.00 D). The latter finding supports the clinical impression that plus lenses lose power when placed upon the eye. Such power changes can therefore account for vision loss during soft lens wear.

Astigmatic Error

An uncorrected astigmatic component of a refraction measured with the contact lens in place may be caused by:
- Astigmatic shift in the refraction of the eye
- Residual uncorrected astigmatism
- Mislocation of a toric lens
- Incorrect lens ordered
- Incorrect lens supplied
- Corneal warpage

Tables are available that allow reconciliation of axis mislocation, cylindrical power of the lens, and resultant refractive error.[10] Again, a full refractive evaluation and checking of lens power is required to ascertain the exact source of the uncorrected astigmatism and allow appropriate action to be taken. Practitioners also should bear in mind the possibility of flexure effects on the eye. Failure of a hydrogel lens to fully align with a toric cornea can lead to a small astigmatic tear lens.[11]

Presbyopia

Middle-aged and elderly contact lens wearers will inevitably have difficulty with near vision unless additional strategies are employed. Aside from using reading spectacles in conjunction with contact lenses for distance vision, contact lens correction of presbyopia entails a variety of visual compromises:

CLINICAL PEARL

Middle-aged and elderly contact lens wearers will inevitably have difficulty with near vision unless additional strategies are employed.

- Monovision. Despite being the most favored alternative, monovision leads to degradation of binocular vision because of the interocular rivalry of clear and blurred images.[12]
- Alternating vision bifocal contact lenses. Incomplete lens translation across the cornea may result in the failure of the desired portion of the lens to cover the pupil.[13]
- Simultaneous vision bifocal contact lenses. At any one time, the retina of each eye will receive both clear and blurred images of the object of interest. The satisfactory performance of such lenses depends on the pupil being large enough to encompass both distance and near portions.[14] Because of poor low-contrast and low-illumination acuities

for higher add powers, Cox et al[15] suggest that simultaneous vision lenses may not be the optimal form of vision correction for older presbyopic patients.

Lens Factors

Problems relating to incorrect lens power were discussed earlier. However, numerous nonoptical factors will influence vision quality with soft contact lenses.

Lens Parameters

Excessive departure from an optimal fit can result in visual degradation. Lenses that are too flat will decenter from the cornea to the point that the optic zone does not cover the pupil. Steep lenses will tend to buckle, creating an uneven optical surface causing degraded and fluctuating vision. Although an optimal fit is generally regarded as necessary for adequate visual performance, research trials have failed to show that fittings 0.3 mm flatter or steeper than optimum influenced vision.[4]

The contrast sensitivity function with higher water content lenses has been measured by Nowozyckyj et al[4] as statistically significantly reduced compared to that with low water content lenses. The reduction was small in magnitude, leading the authors to suggest that the finding may have little clinical relevance. High water content hydrogel lenses that display considerable levels of in-eye dehydration may induce vision loss by inducing epithelial desiccation.[16]

In terms of the mechanical stability of a soft lens on the eye, neither lens thickness nor diameter (at least within commonly accepted clinical bounds) appears to be an important variable in determining visual performance. Physiologically, lenses of increased thickness can have a profound effect on vision by impeding oxygen flow to the cornea and inducing significant edema or other forms of ocular pathology. Such mechanisms are discussed later in this chapter.

Surface Quality

Determination of the optical quality of hydrogel lenses both in vivo and in vitro is difficult. In vivo, the smoothness of the tear layer following a blink can mask an inferior optical surface, whereas the lens' flexibility in vitro provides a barrier to accurate assessment of optical characteristics. The most economical method of determining whether an inferior optical quality of a lens is responsible for decreased vision is to try another lens of the same parameters on the eye.

Deposits

Surface build-up on contact lenses has been clinically associated with reduced visual acuity. A decrease of two to three lines of Snellen acuity over several months of lens wear was reported by McClure et al[17]; however, their results were not analyzed statistically.

Gellatly et al.[18] assessed the visual performance of 51 patients wearing hydroxyethyl methacrylate (HEMA) lenses to establish a relationship among lens deposition, aging, and vision. The study shows that logMAR acuity decreases with increasing lens deposition. Both high- and low-contrast acuity show similar levels of decrease (Figure 6-2). Deposits that were graded as level 1 or 2 on the Rudko deposit classification scale[19] provide comparable acuity; however, a mean loss of approximately a half line with each increasing deposition beyond grade 2 was found. Lens deposition is clearly related to the age of the lens.

Lens Age

Although a relationship exists between lens age and vision (Figure 6-3), this relationship is probably casual rather than causal; the link between the two variables is lens deposition. No direct evidence exists linking age-related polymer degradation to visual decrement.

Total wearing time, rather than the length of time since wear was initiated, determines deposit accumulation on a hydrogel lens.[18] In the

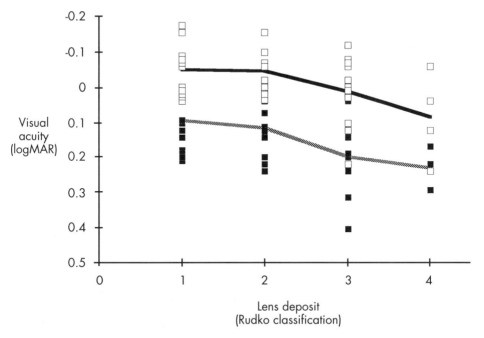

FIGURE 6-2 Relation between visual acuity (logMAR) and the degree of lens deposition (Rudko classification). Data for high-contrast acuity are given by the open boxes and solid line, and data for low-contrast acuity are given by the closed boxes and shaded line. (From Gellatly et al: Visual decrement with deposit accumulation on HEMA contact lenses, *Am J Optom Physiol Optics* 65:937-941, 1988.)

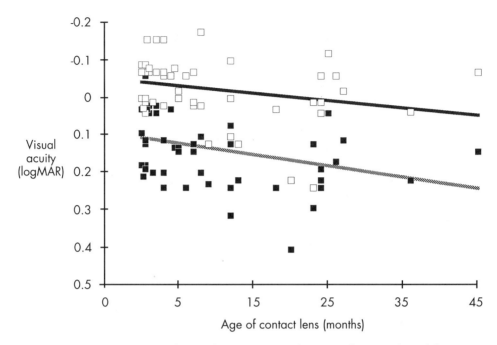

FIGURE 6-3 Relation between visual acuity (logMAR) and lens age (months). Data for high-contrast acuity are given by the open boxes and solid line, and data for low-contrast acuity are given by the closed boxes and shaded line. (From Gellatly et al: Visual decrement with deposit accumulation on HEMA contact lenses, *Am J Optom Physiol Optics* 65:937-941, 1988).

study of Gellatly et al.,[18] only 3% (1 out of 31) of patients whose lenses had been worn for an estimated 2600 hours or less showed a deposit classification of greater than grade 2, whereas 80% (16 out of 20) of patients whose lenses were older than 2600 hours showed this degree of deposition. Because a deposit level of grade 2 appears to be the cut-off for decrease in both high- and low-contrast vision, 2600 hours is recommended as a maximum wearing time for any HEMA lens. This time scale is equivalent to 6 months of full-time daily wear, or 1 year of wear for 10 hours per day, 5 days per week.

Gellatly et al.[18] have outlined a simple clinical protocol for investigating vision loss associated with deposit formation. First, verify the existence of the visual decrement. Assuming no refractive basis can be found for the vision reduction, assess the deposition on the lens. If the deposit grading accounts for the visual decrement, as shown in Figure 6-2, lens replacement is indicated. Rapid lens deposition and concomitant loss of vision may necessitate a regular planned replacement or a disposable lens system. Should the grading not account for the visual decrement, the other possible causes of vision loss (such as ocular pathology) should be sought.[18]

Lens Movement

Transient fluctuation in vision following a blink is one reason patients complain that vision with soft lenses is more variable and of poorer quality compared to that with spectacles. Ridder and Tomlinson[20] found that vision with soft lenses was considerably degraded when a target was presented less than 100 msec after the blink. They explained their finding in terms of blink suppression and prismatic shift of the retinal image induced by the movement of the contact lens produced by the blink. Loose-fitting contact lenses caused an even greater decrement in immediate postblink vision.

CLINICAL PEARL

Transient fluctuation in vision following a blink is one reason patients complain that vision with soft lenses is more variable and of poorer quality compared to that with spectacles.

Eye Factors

The optical quality of the cornea depends on its shape and transparency. These requirements for good vision may be disturbed by the physiological impact of a contact lens, which may cause corneal distortion or result in pathophysiological changes in the various layers of the cornea that interfere with passage of light to the retina.

Infection

The most severe problem accompanying contact lens wear is infectious keratitis. The dense infiltration and corneal edema that accompany the resulting ulcer can seriously affect vision, causing haziness and photophobia. Although several lines of visual acuity may be lost while the infection is active, less severe cases or peripheral corneal infections will result in minimal ultimate visual loss. Serious infections may lead to inflammation and scarring of the infection site, which can result in permanent vision loss. Central infections have caused visual acuity to fall to less than 20/300.[21]

CLINICAL PEARL

Although several lines of visual acuity may be lost while the infection is active, less severe cases or peripheral corneal infections will result in minimal ultimate visual loss.

Quick, accurate diagnosis is vital for the well-being of the patient and preservation of normal vision. Accompanying symptoms and biomicroscopic examination will quickly lead the practitioner to provide therapeutic management in cases of infectious keratitis. Lens wear should be ceased; the primary aim is to prevent permanent vision loss. Only after complete resolution of the infection should lens wear be reconsidered.

Edema

Because the optical clarity of the cornea depends on its state of deturgescence, a decrease in visual performance might be expected in association with corneal edema; however, the low levels of stromal edema observed with daily wear of hydrogel lenses do not affect vision. Overnight lens wear can lead to greater stromal edema (between 10% and 20%),[22] and the patient will notice haze, reduced acuity, and glare sensitivity upon waking. These symptoms last less than 1 hour after eye opening as edema subsides. Bruce[23] measured the effect of closed-eye lens wear on visual acuity with high- and low-contrast vision charts. He demonstrated that stromal edema of 10% leads to an average reduction of visual acuity of approximately one half to one line, for the high- and low-contrast charts respectively.

The mechanism of visual disturbance following overnight contact lens wear does not necessarily relate to light scattering by the stroma; rather, epithelial edema is more likely to accompany high levels of stromal edema. Moderate stromal edema of 9% caused by anoxia has no measurable effect on vision, apart from a minimal decrease in the higher spatial frequencies of contrast sensitivity.[8] Conversely, osmotically induced edema (in which the stroma thickens by only 7%) leads to a marked reduction at all frequencies of contrast sensitivity.[8] The mechanism for osmotically induced vision loss is most likely intercellular epithelial edema. The major symptoms experienced with epithelial edema are haze, glare sensitivity, or the perception of halos around lights. Therefore, contact lenses are only likely to influence vision when epithelial edema is induced, such as with high levels of stromal edema or excessive tearing that occurs during adaptation to lens wear.[24]

Epithelial Disturbance

Interaction between the contact lens and cornea can result in disruption to the superficial layer of epithelial cells, which is observed clinically as epithelial staining following instillation of fluorescein. Extensive staining may be associated with vision reduction because the regular smooth refracting surface of the cornea has been disturbed. A disruption to the superficial epithelium can result from desiccation, eruption of microcysts, solution toxicity, allergic reactions, the presence of a foreign body under the lens, and gross physiological insult (such as hypoxia or hypercapnia). The extent of visual loss is difficult to predict from the clinical presentation of the condition, but generally does not exceed two lines of Snellen acuity.

A considerable amount of vision may be lost with combinations of high water content contact lens materials and lens solution preservatives. In an experimental trial (Brennan, unpublished data) of a high water content material with a quaternary ammonium preservative, all patients using the combination developed visual disturbance some 5 days after beginning lens wear, which progressively worsened (in some cases to less than 20/100) over the following days. Vision remained disturbed for hours following lens removal. Biomicroscopic examination revealed widespread punctate corneal staining. Comfort was unaffected by the condition; indeed, the corneas were anesthetic to the touch of cotton thread. The vision loss in this case is presumed to be caused by severe epithelial edema produced by a toxic reaction to the preservative that remained in the lens.

Vascularization

Severe stromal vascularization as a result of contact lens wear may lead to vision loss. Although asymptomatic in most cases, vascularization can proceed until the central cornea (and thus vision) is affected.[25]

The fibrous nature of the vascular ingrowth can cause permanent opacification of the affected cornea. Many theories about the etiology of stromal vascularization have been advanced, and hypoxia is strongly implicated.[25]

Careful aftercare of contact lens patients is necessary to detect and arrest vessel ingrowth. Substantial development of vessels that pose a threat to vision should lead to cessation of lens wear and perhaps refitting with rigid gas-permeable lenses or hydrogel lenses of greater oxygen permeability.

Infiltrates

Corneal infiltrates are occasionally observed in the stroma in conjunction with a variety of contact–lens-induced pathological states such as infection, acute red eye (noninfectious keratitis), vascularization, and superior limbic keratoconjunctivitis. Infiltrates appear as gray, hazy areas consisting of localized edema and inflammatory cells.[26] Because infiltrates are a form of media opacification, they will interfere with the passage of light through the cornea when they lie in the pupillary zone; however, contact–lens-induced corneal infiltration typically occurs toward the limbus and rarely poses a threat to vision. Treatment strategies should be directed toward removing the stimulus to infiltration, and may involve interruption of lens wear, change of lens design, or switching of lens maintenance systems.

Tear Dysfunction

The tear layer is an important component of the human optical system. Although disruption to this layer will primarily affect comfort, it also may result in a degraded visual image. Improper tear formation on the surface of a contact lens can be attributed to the following factors:

- Hydrophobicity of the lens surface, which is primarily a function of the polymer chemistry; increasing the proportion of methacrylic acid in the lens material renders the lens surface more hydrophilic and improves wetting.
- Lens surface deposition that disrupts the uniform tear film surface tension across the lens, and leads to isolated break-up of the tear film.
- Surface abnormalities such as poorly finished lens surfaces and cracks caused by polymer degradation.
- Incomplete blinking caused by the stimulus to blinking being removed because of the protective effect of the lens on the cornea. This results in the failure of the tears to be spread over the surface of the lens. This is particularly evident during tasks that demand concentration, such as reading.
- Environmental extremes such as in air-conditioned offices or in arid or arctic environments where extremes of temperature and humidity lead to increased evaporation of the aqueous component of the tears.
- Deficiencies of tear quantity or quality that may not become obvious until the lens is worn; in this instance, lens wear is a provocative test of tear function.

Patients with ocular pathological states that result in the incomplete formation of the precorneal tear layer (such as with keratoconjunctivitis sicca) will be particularly prone to vision problems with contact lens wear.

The best type of soft lens for the patient who is susceptible to dry eye is open to debate. Based on their extensive lens dehydration studies, Efron and Brennan[27] have suggested that a lens made from a high water content material with a low free-to-bound water ratio (such as collagen)[28] may be the most suitable.

Shape Changes

Changes in corneal shape during hydrogel lens wear are not as dramatic as changes in response to polymethyl methacrylate (PMMA) lenses, which degrade vision by inducing spectacle blur and corneal warpage. Short-term edema produced by soft lenses is less localized than the central edema of PMMA lens wear, and corneal curvature is relatively unaffected. Furthermore, edema is generally restricted to low values because of the oxygen permeability of hydrogels.

Long-term chronic hypoxia may lead to corneal warpage in hydrogel lens wearers. The phenomenon has been termed corneal exhaustion syndrome.[29] In particular, wearers of thick, high powered, low water content lenses of low oxygen transmissibility appear to be at risk. Changes in corneal shape and stromal thinning[30] accompanied by fluctuating refraction and irregular astigmatism in long-term hydrogel lens wearers should be investigated for the effects of chronic hypoxia. Refitting with rigid gas-permeable lenses allows improved oxygenation while maintaining adequate vision.

Several cases of marked visual disturbance have been reported in which contact lens wear has produced corneal wrinkling. Lowe and Brennan[31] reported on a lens that induced corneal wrinkling in a number of experimental subjects. Vision loss was marked, with a decrease as great as 6/120. The lens was thin, made from a medium water content material, and seemed free of any defects. The corneal deformation was extraordinary, as demonstrated by photokeratoscopy, with the mires showing a 'crinkled' pattern. Other isolated cases of corneal wrinkling have been reported with hard lens wear.[32,33]

Although marked corneal deformation causing major visual disturbance such as that reported by Lowe and Brennan[30] is uncommon, their findings can explain vision loss in some patients if no other mechanism has been isolated. Indeed, it is possible that a low-grade corneal deformity occurs in these patients. Clinical investigation of mild corneal warpage is difficult because biomicroscopic observation provides little information about corneal shape change, and the information provided by keratometry pertains solely to the central cornea.

Binocular Vision

The different demands on accommodation and convergence with contact lenses, as compared to spectacles frequently result in asthenopic symptoms in patients undertaking near vision tasks during contact lens wear. In particular, the myopic individual will experience a lesser demand on accommodation and a greater demand on convergence during near work, which stresses the accommodation/convergence synkinesis. The inability of the patient to adapt to the new binocular demands may necessitate supplementary binocular vision treatment.

Conclusion

The wide-ranging subjective appreciation of vision reported by patients wearing hydrogel lenses does not always correlate with recorded visual acuity. Some patients with poor acuity are satisfied with their vision, whereas others who complain of visual difficulties with their contact lenses exhibit normal acuity. Possible explanations of this phenomenon include psychological factors, wherein motivation arising from the cosmetic advantages of contact lenses overrides visual considerations, and inadequacy of methods for testing visual function.

This chapter has presented an overview of factors that can lead to vision loss during soft contact lens wear, and has proposed clinical strategies for determining its cause when it is not obvious. A summary of the major causes of vision loss associated with soft contact lens wear is presented in Figure 6-4.

Characterization of Vision Loss

	Immediate	Severe	Fluctuating	Without lens	Near	Haze	Glare
Uncorrected refraction	√	?			?		
Decentered lens	√	?	√				
Loss of lens	√	?			?		
Toric misalignment	√		?		√		
Lens deposits			?			√	√
Infectious keratitis	√	?		√	√	?	√
Stromal edema							?
Epithelial edema		?		√		√	√
Toxic/Allergic		?		√	?	√	?
Tear film abnormality	?		√	?	√	?	
Altered corneal shape		?		√	√		
Binocular vision	?		√		√		

FIGURE 6-4 Summary of lens and eye factors (rows) causing various types of vision loss (columns). Eye factors are defined as **immediate** (vision loss noticed immediately upon lens insertion), **severe** (severe vision loss), **fluctuating** (fluctuating vision during wear), **without lens** (vision reduced immediately following lens removal), **near** (vision reduced at near), **haze** (hazy vision), and **glare** (glare symptoms). A checkmark signifies a strong association; a question mark signifies a possible association.

References

1. Woo G, Hess RF: Contrast sensitivity function and soft contact lenses, *Int Cont Lens Clin* 6:171-176, 1979.
2. Grey CP: Changes in contrast sensitivity during the first week of soft contact lens wear, *Am J Optom Physiol Opt* 64:768-774, 1987.
3. Teitelbaum BA, Kelly SA, Gemoules G: Contrast sensitivity through spectacles and hydrogel lenses of different polymers, *Int Cont Lens Clin* 12:162-166, 1985.
4. Nowozyckyj A, Carney LG, Efron N: Effect of hydrogel lens wear on contrast sensitivity, *Am J Optom Physiol Opt* 65:263-271, 1988.
5. Tomlinson A, Mann G: An analysis of visual performance with contact lens and spectacle correction, *Ophthalmol Physiol Opt* 5:53-57, 1985.
6. Guillon M, Lydon DPM, Solman RT: Effect of target contrast and luminance on soft contact lens and spectacle visual performance, *Curr Eye Res* 7:635-648, 1988.
7. Bailey IL, Lovie JE: New design principles for visual acuity letter charts, *Am J Optom Physiol Opt* 53:740-745, 1976.
8. Carney LG, Jacobs RJ: Mechanisms of visual loss in corneal edema, *Arch Ophthalmol* 102:1068-1071, 1984.
9. Weissman BA: A general relation between changing surface radii of flexing soft contact lenses, *Am J Optom Physiol Opt* 61:651-653, 1984.
10. Dain SJ: Overrefraction and axis mislocation of toric lenses, *Int Cont Lens Clin* 6:86-90, 1979.
11. Weissman BA, Gardner KM: Flexure effects of double-thin zone toric soft contact lenses, *Am J Optom Physiol Opt* 61:465-468, 1984.
12. Sheedy JE, Harris MG, Busby L, Chan E, Coga I: Monovision contact lens wear and occupational task performance, *Am J Optom Physiol Opt* 65:14-18, 1988.
13. Robboy M, Erickson P: Performance comparison of current hydrophilic alternating vision bifocal contact lenses, *Int Cont Lens Clin* 14:237-243, 1987.
14. McGill E, Ames K, Erickson P, Robboy M: Quality of vision with hydrogel simultaneous vision bifocal contact lenses, *Int Cont Lens Clin* 14:476-481, 1987.
15. Cox I, Ames K, Apollonio A, Erickson P: The effect of add power on simultaneous vision, monocentric, bifocal, soft lenses visual performance, *Int Cont Lens Clin* 20:18-21, 1993.
16. Holden BA, Sweeney DF, Seger RG: Epithelial erosions caused by thin high water content lenses, *Clin Exp Optom* 69:103-107, 1986.
17. McClure DA, Ohota S, Eriksen SP, Randeri KJ: The effect on measured visual acuity of protein deposition and removal in soft contact lenses, *Contacto* 21:8-12, 1977.
18. Gellatly KW, Brennan NA, Efron N: Visual decrement with deposit accumulation on HEMA contact lenses, *Am J Optom Physiol Opt* 65:937-941, 1988.
19. Rudko P, Proby J: A method for classifying and describing protein deposition on the hydrophilic contact lens, *Allergen Report Series* 94, 1974.
20. Ridder WH, Tomlinson A: Blink-induced, temporal variations in contrast sensitivity, *Int Cont Lens Clin* 18:231-237, 1991.
21. Brennan NA: Current thoughts on the etiology of ocular changes during contact lens wear, *Aust J Optom* 68:8-24, 1985.
22. LaHood D, Sweeney DF, Holden BA: Overnight corneal edema with hydrogel, rigid gas permeable and silicone elastomer contact lenses, *Int Cont Lens Clin* 15:149-154, 1988.
23. Bruce AS: Assessment of corneal function during extended wear of hydrogel contact lenses, PhD thesis, University of Melbourne, 1991.
24. Cox I, Holden BA: Can vision loss be used as a quantitative assessment of corneal edema? *Int Cont Lens Clin* 17:176-180, 1990.
25. Efron N: Contact lens-induced corneal neovascularisation, *Optician* 211(5533):26-35, 1996.
26. Zantos SG: Management of corneal infiltrates in extended-wear contact lens patients, *Int Cont Lens Clin* 11:604-610, 1984.

27. Efron N, Brennan NA: The clinical relevance of hydrogel lens water content, *Trans Br Cont Lens Assoc Ann Clin Conf* 4:9-14, 1987.
28. Efron N, Young G: Dehydration of hydrogel lenses in vitro and in vivo, *Ophthalmol Physiol Opt* 8:253-256, 1988.
29. Sweeney DF: Corneal exhaustion syndrome with long-term wear of contact lenses, *Optom Vis Sci* 69:601-608, 1992.
30. Holden BA, Sweeney DF, Vannas A, Nilsson KT, Efron N: Effects of long-term extended contact lens wear on the human cornea, *Inv Ophthalmol Vis Sci* 26:1489-1501, 1985.
31. Lowe R, Brennan NA: Corneal wrinkling caused by a thin medium water content lens, *Int Cont Lens Clin* 14:403-406, 1987.
32. Quinn TG: Epithelial folds, *Int Cont Lens Clin* 9:365, 1982.
33. Rosenthal JW: Corneal wrinkling with contact lenses, *Am J Ophthalmol* 55:138-139, 1963.

7

Comfort Problems with Contact Lenses

Nathan Efron
Noel A. Brennan

Key Terms

contact lens	analog grading	anterior ocular
soft lens	scale	tissues

The most common symptom a contact lens practitioner will confront is discomfort. Reconciliation of patient symptoms with clinical signs is a constant challenge to health care practitioners. The potential always exists to devote undue attention to a complaint that bears little significance to the patient's well-being or, conversely, to give token consideration to a symptom arising from a potentially serious condition. Furthermore, many signs that the clinician detects will have a major influence on patient management, but the patient will show few or no symptoms. Conditions that may be asymptomatic such as corneal vascularization, microcystic edema, and endothelial polymegethism are important pathophysiological signs that require some form of treatment. However, the most rewarding management plans, from the perspective of the patient, are those that alleviate discomfort.

During adaptation to contact lens wear, soft lenses offer greater comfort than rigid lenses. Indeed, a study that assessed hydrogel lens

This chapter has been reproduced from Efron N, Brennan NA, How to manage complaints of discomfort during contact lens wear (Ch.2), in *The International Contact Lens Year Book*, (Ed) N. Efron, Saunders, 1993, pp. 7-20.

comfort over short wearing periods found that more than half of lens wearers were unaware of the presence of the lens in their eyes at any given moment.[1] Both soft and rigid lenses are comfortable once the patient has adapted to them. Nonetheless, occasions will arise when lenses become uncomfortable. Because of the subjective nature of discomfort symptoms, most reports in the literature concerning this topic have been anecdotal. In this chapter, an attempt will be made to bring together results of analytical studies to give a scientific basis to the phenomenon of ocular sensation during contact lens wear. Management plans for solving the various problems will be suggested.

Defining and Measuring Discomfort

Categories of Symptoms

Patients wearing contact lenses commonly report that their eyes feel scratchy, dry, watery, itchy, gritty, hot, or burning; they also may use less specific terms such as tired, irritated, uncomfortable, or sore.

Dryness seems to be the most frequently occurring symptom (Figure 7-1). In a survey of 104 patients wearing HEMA contact lenses, Brennan and Efron[2] found that 75% of patients experience dryness at times, although less than 20% of patients report that this occurs often. This compares to 52% who notice that their eyes feel

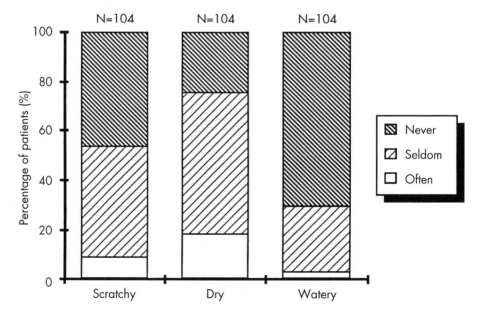

FIGURE 7-1 Frequency with which a sample group of patients wearing HEMA lenses complained of the symptoms scratchy, dry, and watery. (From Brennan NA, Efron, N: Symtomatology of HEMA lens wearers, *Optom Vis Sci* 66:834-838, 1989.)

scratchy at times, and 30% who notice that their eyes feel watery at times.[2] McMonnies and Ho also have found dryness to be the most frequently reported symptom among soft lens wearers.[3]

Quantifying Discomfort

The scientific assessment of comfort relating to contact lens wear poses a number of problems common to other fields that investigate subjective responses to a stimulus. Comfort responses to contact lens wear can be assessed using the following techniques, which are ranked in order of increasing sophistication and power:

Nominal—in which a specific severity of a specific sensation can be purely descriptive. For example, the terms "painless," "no sensation," "moderate pain," and "severe discomfort" could be used.

Ordinal—in which a specific sensation can be ranked on a numerical scale with discrete stages of severity, such as grade 0, 1, 2, or 3.

Analog—in which a specific sensation can be ranked on a continuous scale; the subject indicates the relative comfort level by placing a mark anywhere on a line upon which are gross indicators of the degree of comfort. The distance from one end of the line to the mark is measured and taken as an index of the magnitude of the sensation. The analog scale is usually presented vertically to remove possible effects of handedness (Figure 7-2).

The analog technique is the most powerful because it allows parametric statistics to be used on the data, based on the assumption of normal distribution of error in the position of the marked response. Even where the assumption of normality is invalid, a more rigorous nonparametric analysis may be effected.

Avoiding Bias When Measuring Discomfort

General strategies that are employed in scientific investigation to minimize the effects of experimenter and subject bias are particularly relevant to the assessment of subjective responses to contact lens wear. These include masking, randomization, and the use of experimental controls. One procedure that has been adopted in such experiments is to elicit a response from subjects using a printed card to avoid possible bias that could be introduced by inappropriate voice intonations associated with verbal prompting.[1] In conducting contact lens trials, a difficult problem to avoid is the strong preconceptions of the experimental subjects of the advantages and disadvantages of contact lenses.

CLINICAL PEARL

In conducting contact lens trials, a difficult problem to avoid is the strong preconceptions of the experimental subjects of the advantages and disadvantages of contact lenses.

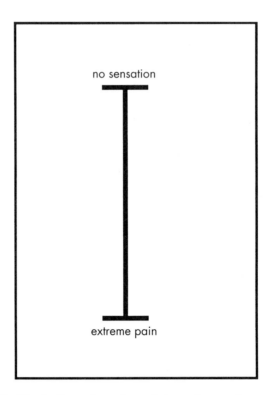

FIGURE 7-2 Vertically oriented analog scale used to measure the degree of discomfort. The subject is asked to place a mark across the scale at a level that indicates the level of discomfort.

Determining Whether Discomfort is Lens Related or Eye Related

Certain strategies may be employed to determine whether the source of discomfort is related to the lens or the eye:

Concurrent ocular pathology—The possibility that discomfort during lens wear is caused by concurrent ocular pathology unrelated to lens wear should not be overlooked. Practitioners should always be prepared to conduct additional tests to exclude the possibility of extraneous pathology.

Laterality—The laterality of a condition is often of diagnostic significance. For example, a toxicity reaction to preservatives in disinfecting solutions would produce discomfort and redness in both eyes, whereas discomfort caused by a lens defect is likely to produce discomfort only in the affected eye.

Lens removal—If discomfort persists for a considerable time after lens removal, then it is likely that the ocular tissues have been compromised. Immediate relief following lens removal suggests a lens defect, although a foreign body beneath the lens may have been the cause of discomfort. Recurrence of discomfort in an otherwise quiet eye after reintroduction of a lens clearly points toward a lens defect.

Lens swap between eyes—If a patient is experiencing unexplained discomfort in one eye during lens wear, the lenses should be removed and placed in the opposite eyes. Following this swap, discomfort in the same eye indicates an eye-related problem, whereas transference of the discomfort to the other eye indicates a lens-related problem.

Ocular lubricants—Instillation of an ocular lubricant into an uncomfortable lens-wearing eye may provide relief; this would indicate a mechanical or abrasive source of discomfort.

Physiological Explanations of Discomfort

Adaptation

Upon wear of hydrogel lenses for the first time, the patient experiences heightened lens awareness, a phenomenon that is particularly acute with rigid lenses. As a result, lens wear on the first day is generally restricted to a few hours, and is increased 1 or 2 hours per day until the desired wearing time is achieved. The physiological basis for adaptation to contact lens wear is poorly understood.

Neural Sensation

The neural mechanisms by which the conjunctiva and cornea produce ocular sensations during contact lens wear have yet to be elucidated. Certainly these mechanisms are somewhat imprecise. For example, ocular sensations are often so poorly differentiated that a description and localization of an abnormal ocular event by a patient are often inaccurate. It is therefore not surprising that patient reports of ocular sensations can be confusing to the practitioner. In the absence of major lens or eye anomalies, the comfort of the lens appears to depend upon the interaction between the lid and lens.

The nature of the stimulus that causes dryness also is unclear, and the reasons for the high frequency of this symptom in contact lens wearers are a matter for speculation; it is the least frequently reported symptom of nonwearers.[3] Because there are no specific "dryness receptors" in human tissue, ocular dryness must be a response to specific coding of afferent neural inputs. One may hypothesize that dryness results from an interference with tear physiology and structure by the contact lens, the specific mechanism being increased tear evaporation and faster break-up of the tear film. The sensation also may arise from the neural misinterpretation of stimuli seemingly unrelated to dryness, such as direct mechanical interaction of the lens with the ocular tissues, lens dehydration, or vasodilation and the subsequent rise in local temperature.

CLINICAL PEARL

Because there are no specific "dryness receptors" in human tissue, ocular dryness must be a response to specific coding of afferent neural inputs.

Lens Factors

General Considerations

Some of the more common and easily solved problems that can lead to discomfort include:
- Poor fitting lenses
- Physical defects in lenses
- Particulate matter partially embedded in lens surfaces
- Foreign bodies beneath lenses

Other major lens-related causes of discomfort include inappropriate lens design, dehydration, aging, deposit-related irritation, and lens imperfections.

Lens Design

That thin, rounded lens edges provide greater comfort than thicker, square edges was recognized by the pioneers of contact lens practice a century ago.[4,5] Most contact lens clinicians today would agree that the edge design of any contact lens is a key variable in determining comfort. Guidelines for the optimization of the edge design of contact lenses have been provided by a number of authors.[6-8]

CLINICAL PEARL

Most contact lens clinicians today would agree that the edge design of any contact lens is a key variable in determining comfort.

The interrelationship of lens thickness and water content is an important consideration in the design of hydrogel lenses that also has a bearing on lens comfort. Although high water lenses may be more comfortable in the long term,[9] lenses manufactured from high water content materials are initially less comfortable than lenses manufactured from low water content materials[1] because higher water content lenses must be made thicker for purposes of mechanical resilience. A thicker lens has a greater mechanical effect in the eye and contributes to a higher degree of initial lens awareness.[1] It is generally held that thinner lenses are more comfortable.[10-12]

Brennan and Efron[2] found that 40% of patients wearing toric HEMA lenses reported often experiencing dryness, whereas only 13%

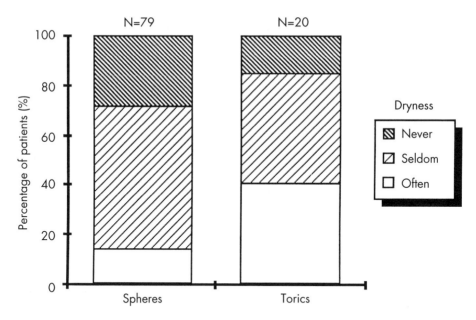

FIGURE 7-3 Frequency with which a sample group of patients wearing spherical and toric HEMA lenses complained of dryness. (From Brennan NA, Efron N: Symptomatology of HEMA lens wearers, *Optom Vis Sci* 66:834-838, 1989.)

of patients wearing spherical lenses reported experiencing this symptom (Figure 7-3). The reason for this finding is unclear, but may be caused by neural misinterpretation of the thick portion of a toric lens.

Other lens design strategies that have been advocated for maximizing lens comfort include decreasing lens movement[13] and increasing lens diameter.[14]

Dehydration

Dryness during HEMA lens wear has been correlated with the amount of dehydration the lenses show on the eye.[15] The water content of lenses worn by patients who report that their eyes often feel dry during lens wear is reduced compared to that of patients who never experience this symptom (Figure 7-4). It is likely that the cause of dryness and the measurable change in lens water content is related to a deficient tear film.

Lens Age and Deposit Formation

Older lenses are associated with an increased frequency of dryness (Figure 7-5). In the Brennan-Efron survey of HEMA lens wearers, 31% of patients with lenses older than 6 months reported experiencing dryness often, compared to only 12% of patients whose lenses were

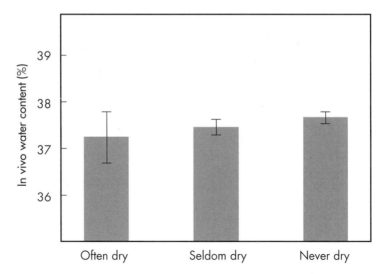

FIGURE 7-4 Mean in vivo water content of patients who reported dryness often (N = 19), seldom (N = 59), and never (N = 26). (From Efron N, Brennan NA: A survey of wearers of low water content hydrogel contact lenses, *Clin Exp Optom* 71:86-90, 1988.)

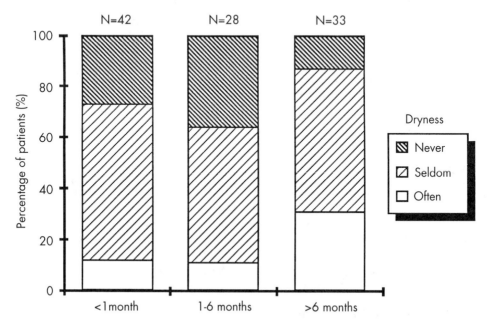

FIGURE 7-5 Frequency with which a sample group of patients wearing HEMA lenses of various ages complained of dryness. (From Brennan NA, Efron N: Symtomatology of HEMA lens wearers, *Optom Vis Sci* 66:834-838, 1989.)

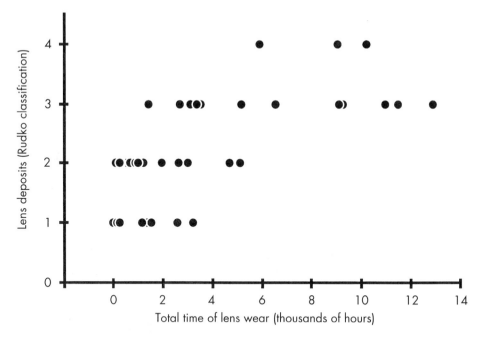

FIGURE 7-6 Relation between lens deposition (Rudko classification) and total time of lens wear in thousands of hours. (From Gellatly KW, Brennan NA, Efron N: Visual decrement with deposit accumulation on HEMA contact lenses, *Am J Optom Physiol Opt* 65:937-941, 1988.)

less than 6 months old.[2] This finding is not surprising given the increased surface build-up following 6 months of wear reported by Gellatly et al (Figure 7-6).[16] Efron and Brennan were unable to demonstrate a change in water content with aging, suggesting that hydrogel lens dehydration does not contribute to the age-related decrease in comfort.[15]

Lens Imperfections

The normally smooth surface of a hydrogel lens, buffered by the multilayered precorneal tear film, offers a mild mechanical stimulus to which the patient readily adapts. A poorly finished lens surface caused by incomplete or improper manufacture and polishing can irritate the adjacent corneal and conjunctival surfaces, causing considerable discomfort. Imperfections on the surface or edge of a lens are usually detected at the delivery visit. This is not the case with disposable lenses, which are dispensed (via the practitioner) from the manufacturer directly to the patient. Defect-related discomfort in its milder form may be masked by the lens awareness typically experienced in the early adaptive stages of wear, particularly in first-time lens wearers. Defects that may be found in soft lenses are illustrated in Figure 7-7.

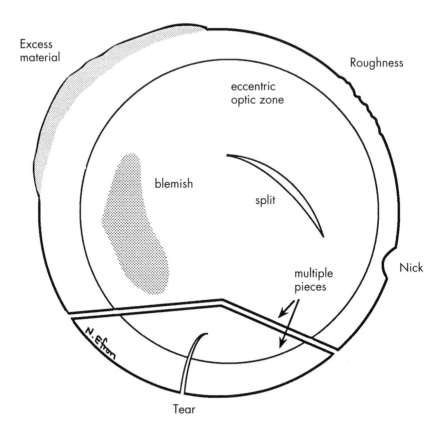

FIGURE 7-7 Schematic representation of types of defects that may be found on soft contact lenses. Captions describing edge and nonedge (body) defects are in upper and lower case, respectively. (From Efron N, Veys J: Defects in disposable contact lenses can compromise ocular integrity, *Int Cont Lens Clin* 19:8-18, 1992.)

A lens that during the course of handling and wear has become torn or chipped, or developed some other surface irregularity, may become uncomfortable. Such defects may be microscopic and could go undetected even under careful examination. A lens should be replaced if the patient persistently complains of irritation and discomfort, even if the specific cause cannot be identified. In the initial period following the fitting of a new lens, contact lens manufacturers are usually agreeable to facilitating such exchanges, particularly if the discomfort was experienced upon initial insertion of the lens.

Microscopic defects in disposable soft lenses do not appear to cause undue discomfort.[17] Indirect evidence that more extensive lens defects will cause greater discomfort comes from a study on soft lens fenestrations by Ang and Efron.[18] Fenestrations in soft lenses (which can be considered deliberately introduced "lens defects") were associated with discomfort, with discomfort increasing with increasing fenestration size.

Eye Factors

Numerous pathophysiological changes can be induced in the ocular tissues by contact lenses, many of which lead to discomfort. Thorough examination with the biomicroscope will usually lead the practitioner to a correct diagnosis for these conditions, which are considered here in relation to the tissues affected.

Pathology of Corneal Epithelium

Interruption to the physical integrity of the corneal epithelium can cause considerable discomfort. The intensity of discomfort, however, is not always directly related to the severity of the epithelial disturbance as assessed with fluorescein. For example, a small foreign body track may be associated with severe pain whereas an exposure keratitis leading to extensive inferior arcuate staining may be asymptomatic.

Patients displaying corneal epithelial microcysts often complain of mild discomfort, although it is not understood whether this is a causal or casual relationship. Severe epithelial edema such as can be induced osmotically in the research laboratory can induce considerable pain, but levels of epithelial edema experienced clinically are generally asymptomatic. Infectious keratitis is frequently associated with extreme pain.

Stromal Edema

Moderate levels of contact–lens-induced edema may be associated with mild discomfort. However, high levels of edema, as may occur if a patient wears a low oxygen transmissibility contact lens overnight, can be associated with extreme discomfort. Under such conditions the edema must not be considered in isolation, because concurrent pathological changes could account for the discomfort, such as conjunctival congestion or a mild anterior uveal response. The same is true for corneal exhaustion syndrome, a term given to an acquired intolerance to lens wear following years of wearing low oxygen transmissibility contact lenses. This syndrome also may be characterized by high levels of edema and endothelial polymegethism.

Infiltrates

Acute red eye is a common cause of ocular discomfort in association with hydrogel lens wear. The condition is characterized by mild to severe pain, photophobia, lacrimation, and conjunctival redness; it often occurs following overnight wear of a hydrogel lens and is usually unilateral. Biomicroscopic examination will typically reveal conjunctival and limbal injection, and a region of stromal infiltration, all of which can be observed adjacent to the site of the keratitis.

Infiltrates are comprised of edema and aggregates of white blood cells that enter the cornea in response to an inflammatory stimulus.[19] The response may be caused by a number of factors including hypoxia, immune response to deposits or solution preservatives, physical irritation, local infection, or inflammation in response to debris trapped beneath the contact lens. Lens removal relieves the immediate stimulus, although the infiltration will frequently remain for over a month. The response may recur, and alteration to lens fit or removal of other potential stimuli is advisable.

Papillary Conjunctivitis

Deposit build-up on lens surfaces can cause mechanical irritation to the eye and initiate an immune reaction. Contact–lens-induced papillary conjunctivitis (CLPC) is a common sequela of these events and is associated with foreign body sensation and general discomfort during lens wear.

CLPC is a common cause of discomfort for hydrogel lens wearers. Increased lens awareness and itching are frequently reported symptoms. Upper lid eversion allows observation of the palpebral conjunctiva, which will display enlarged papillae on the palpebral conjunctival surface. The etiology of CLPC is probably a combined mechanical-immunological mechanism. The rubbing of the lens surface or a rough surface created by deposits on the lens against the palpebral conjunctiva seems to disrupt the conjunctival epithelium. The immunological response may be against denatured protein on the lens surface, solution preservatives used during disinfection that may have become absorbed into the lens matrix, or deposits on the lens surface. The type of deposit and the way the protein adheres to the lens may be important in determining the magnitude of the tissue response.

The acute phase of CLPC should be treated by ceasing lens wear. The papillae may persist for months but contact lens wear may be recommenced, with reduced wearing times, when the acute phase has subsided. Changing to a hydrogen peroxide lens maintenance system, together with more frequent use of enzymatic cleaning systems can give improved results. Refitting with rigid or hydrogel lenses of a different design also may allow lens wear to continue, although recurrence is common.[20]

Superior Limbic Keratoconjunctivitis

Superior limbic keratoconjunctivitis (SLK) occurs almost exclusively in soft lens wearers and may produce increased lens awareness, burning, itching, photophobia, and hazy vision. The condition is characterized by corneal and conjunctival changes under the upper lid. Signs include hyperemia of the superior limbus and adjacent conjunctiva, fibrovascular corneal pannus, and stromal infiltrates. The affected regions of the conjunctiva and cornea may stain with fluorescein.

Although a distinct etiology has yet to be determined, SLK may be caused by local hypoxia under the upper lid, mechanical irritation caused by the lens edge and deposits, or may be an immunological reaction to solution preservatives or denatured protein on the lens surface. Symptoms are alleviated by ceasing lens wear; refitting with rigid lenses or different hydrogels is frequently successful.

Tear Film Dysfunction

The quantity and quality of the tear film are important in determining ocular comfort during lens wear. Contact lens wear itself can produce dry eye symptoms in patients whose tear layers seem normal before lens wear commences. Orsborn and Robboy[21] have shown that inferior tear prism height is reduced in patients who report dryness during lens wear; however, these patients show tear prism heights no different from ultimately successful lens-wearing patients before wear commences.

CLINICAL PEARL

Contact lens wear itself can produce dry eye symptoms in patients whose tear layers seem normal before lens wear commences.

Female patients who use oral contraceptives are more likely to report dry eye symptoms during lens wear. Scratchiness and dryness are reported by 32% and 63% respectively, of women not using oral contraceptives, compared with 73% and 100% respectively of women using oral contraceptives (Figures 7-8 and 7-9). Although the mechanism by which oral contraceptives increase the likelihood of symptoms during lens wear is not understood, it is likely that the tear layer is adversely influenced by hormone use.

Lens lubricants are commonly prescribed to relieve dryness in contact lens wearers. Efron et al have established the efficacy of such solutions for patients wearing soft lenses.[22] However, formulas that have been designed specifically to relieve discomfort were shown to offer performance no different than saline solution. Thus a psychological component to subjective symptom relief cannot be discounted. Furthermore, it was not possible to demonstrate that a decrease in the amount of dehydration of the contact lenses was the cause of improvements in comfort. The instillation of lens lubricants stabilizes the prelens tear film temporarily, but within 5 minutes the tear break-up

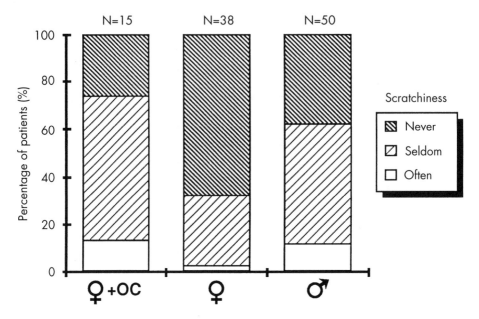

FIGURE 7-8 Frequency of scratchiness for women using oral contraceptives (left bar), women not using oral contraceptives (center bar), and men (right bar) wearing HEMA lenses. (From Brennan NA, Efron N: Symptomatology of HEMA lens wearers, *Optom Vis Sci* 66:834-838, 1989.)

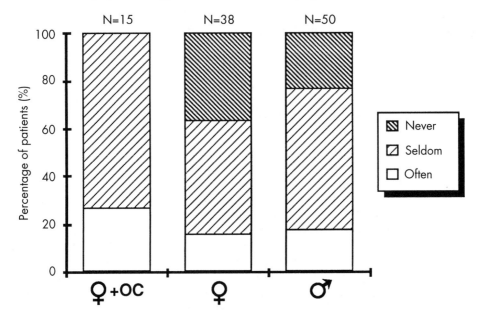

FIGURE 7-9 Frequency of dryness for women using oral contraceptives (left bar), women not using oral contraceptives (center bar) and men (right bar) wearing HEMA lenses. (From Brennan NA, Efron N: Symptomatology of HEMA lens wearers, *Optom Vis Sci* 66:834-838, 1989.)

time is indistinguishable from the preinstillation value.[23] Because the lubricant drops seem to provide relief over a greater period of time, tear film stabilization cannot be proposed as a mechanism of action.

Solution Factors

Solutions used for contact lens maintenance must be compatible with ocular tissues. This requires a compromise, because formulas necessary for effective cleaning or disinfection are often toxic to the eye. Discomfort will result if a lens is introduced into the eye directly from such a solution without intermediate rinsing or neutralization.

Solution pH

Acidity of the soaking solution may lead to discomfort and irritation. Hydrogen peroxide soaking solutions are often buffered to a pH of between 3 and 4; buffered solutions at this pH will cause a major aversion response if placed in the eye.[24]

Solution Tonicity

Most contact lens solution manufacturers formulate their solutions to have a tonicity of 0.9% sodium chloride, which approximates to the salinity of human tears. Contact lenses also are supplied from manufacturers in normal saline. Interestingly, Fletcher and Brennan[25] found that solutions in the range from 0.9% to 2.0% sodium chloride induced the least discomfort, the optimal tonicity being 1.3%. The stinging often reported by patients upon insertion of a hydrogel lens may be at least partially attributable to the tonicity of the lens soaking solution falling outside the optimal range.

Residual Preservatives

One major source of ocular irritation is the introduction into the eye of lens disinfecting solutions. In particular, solution components can enter and become concentrated in the matrix of a soft lens and be released into the eye during subsequent wear. A similar mechanism may occur with respect to lens deposits, which may absorb solution preservatives and release them back into the eye in a more concentrated form. In addition to causing ocular discomfort, the disinfecting agent may initiate a potentially serious toxic or allergic ocular reaction. This problem is being overcome with the increasing availability of disinfecting solutions containing high molecular weight preservatives that are generally too large to be absorbed into the polymer matrix.

Residual Hydrogen Peroxide

The presence of residual hydrogen peroxide within the water component of a hydrogel lens may produce discomfort upon lens insertion, depending on the concentration of the hydrogen peroxide and the integrity of the corneal surface. The most commonly used concentration of hydrogen peroxide in contact lens disinfecting solutions is 3.0%. If a patient omits the neutralization step, insertion of the lens will result in a major reaction characterized by pain, severe stinging, and photophobia. Epithelial staining, injection, and conjunctival chemosis is visible. Within several hours this reaction subsides.

Paugh et al determined that the concentration of hydrogen peroxide required to avoid discomfort was as low as 100 parts per million (ppm).[26] Two subjects in this study who demonstrated apparently minor epithelial defects were extremely sensitive to the lowest concentration of hydrogen peroxide tested, 25 ppm. Because some contact lens disinfecting solutions leave a residual hydrogen peroxide concentration in excess of these levels,[27] it is not surprising that the use of some systems results in a stinging sensation upon lens insertion.

Discomfort usually subsides rapidly following exposure to the low levels of hydrogen peroxide in currently marketed systems; however, discomfort should be noted by the practitioner and used as a sign that neutralization may be inadequate. The answer to the problem of inadequate disinfection may be to change the system or increase neutralization by increasing the time for neutralization or replacing the catalytic disc, whichever is appropriate.

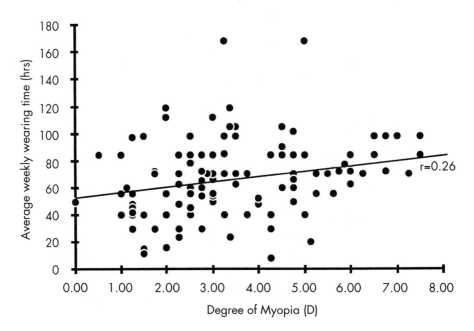

FIGURE 7-10 Number of hours of lens wear per week reported by HEMA lens wearers with various degrees of myopia. (From Efron N, Brennan NA, Sek B: Wearing patterns with HEMA contact lenses, *Int Cont Lens Clin* 15:344-350, 1988.)

Conclusion

Ultimately, patient comfort has a major bearing on the ability to wear contact lenses, and on total wearing time. However, Efron et al[28] were unable to verify this hypothesis. The only factor that correlated with wearing time was the degree of ametropia of the subjects surveyed (Figure 7-10). This suggests that motivation in terms of the poorness of vision without contact lenses is the most important factor regulating wearing activities. An important clinical ramification of this finding is

Characterization of Discomfort

	Immediate	Severe	With blink	Without lens	Scratchy	Dry
Excessive movement	√		√			
Dehydration			?			√
Age and deposits	√	?			?	?
Lens imperfections	√	√	√		√	
Epithelial disruption	√	?	?	?	√	
Foreign body	√	√	√		√	
Edema				?		
CLPC		?	√		?	?
CLSLK		?	√		?	?
Tear film abnormality		?	√			√
Solutions toxicity	?	?				
Solution hypersensitivity		?				

FIGURE 7-11 Summary of lens and eye factors (rows) causing various types of discomfort (columns). The latter are defined as **immediate**—discomfort noticed immediately upon lens insertion; **severe**—severe discomfort; **with blink**—discomfort exacerbated by blinking; **without lens**—discomfort reduced immediately following lens removal; **scratchy**—eye feels scratchy; and **dry**—eye feels dry. A checkmark signifies a strong association; a question mark signifies a possible association.

that patients will not regulate their wearing time according to symptoms alone; this places more of the burden of regulating patient lens wearing habits on the practitioner. Furthermore, the practitioner cannot rely on information about wearing time to determine whether a patient is experiencing major difficulties, and should use criteria such as those discussed in this article to gauge comfort levels.

A summary of the major causes of discomfort associated with contact lens wear is presented in Figure 7-11. Practitioners can use this as a framework to reconcile the various sensations that patients report with observed clinical signs, and as a starting point to develop problem-solving strategies.

The investigation of problems relating to discomfort can be perplexing, but it is extremely rewarding if a solution is found. The broad principles and general problem-solving strategies outlined in this chapter are intended to assist contact lens practitioners in maintaining high levels of patient satisfaction.

References

1. Efron N, Brennan NA, Currie JM, Fitzgerald JP, Hughes MT: Determinants of the initial comfort of hydrogel contact lenses, *Am J Optom Physiol Opt* 63:819-823, 1986.
2. Brennan NA, Efron N: Symptomatology of HEMA lens wearers, *Optom Vis Sci* 66:834-838, 1989.
3. McMonnies CW, Ho A: Marginal dry eye diagnosis: history versus biomicroscopy. In Holly, ed: *The Preocular Tear Film in Health, Disease, and Contact Lens Wear*, Lubbock, 1986, The Dry Eye Institute.
4. Efron N, Pearson RM: Centenary celebration of Fick's Eine Contactbrille, *Arch Ophthalmol* 106:1370-1377, 1988.
5. Pearson RM, Efron N: Hundredth anniversary of August Müllers's inaugural dissertation on contact lenses, *Surv Ophthalmol* 34:133-141, 1989.
6. Hernandez V, Tomlinson A: The effect of soft lens edge thickness, *Cont Lens Forum* 8:77-83, 1983.
7. Smart CFG: The edge forms of contact lenses, *Cont Lens J* 12:5-16, 1984.
8. LaHood D: Edge shape and comfort of rigid lenses, *Am J Optom Physiol Opt* 65:613-618, 1988.
9. Bier N, Lowther GE: *Contact Lens Correction*, London, 1977, Butterworths.
10. Solomon J: An investigation of the ultra-thin Soflens contact lens, *Int Cont Lens Clin* 5:56-60, 1978.
11. Mandell RB: Why are gel lenses more comfortable?, *Int Cont Lens Clin* 1:30-31, 1974.
12. Jurkus JM, Schwartz CA: Ultra-thin hydrophilic lenses: a "comfort study," *Cont Lens Forum* 8:75-83, 1983.
13. Mandell RB: *Contact Lens Practice*, Springfield, Illinois, 1988, Charles C Thomas.
14. Callender M: An evaluation of Bausch and Lomb ultra-thin Soflens (polymacon) contact lenses, *Can J Optom* 41:79-82, 1979.
15. Efron N, Brennan NA: A survey of wearers of low water content hydrogel contact lenses, *Clin Exp Optom* 71:86-90, 1988.
16. Gellatly KW, Brennan NA, Efron N: Visual decrement with deposit accumulation on HEMA contact lenses, *Am J Optom Physiol Opt* 65:937-941, 1988.
17. Efron N, Veys J: Defects in disposable contact lenses can compromise ocular integrity, *Int Cont Lens Clin* 19:8-18, 1992.
18. Ang JHB, Efron N: Comfort of fenestrated hydrogel lenses, *Clin Exp Optom* 70:117-120, 1987.

19. Efron N, Holden BA: A review of some common contact lens complications. Part 1: The corneal epithelium and stroma, *Optician* 192:21-26, 1986.
20. Donshik PC, Ballow M, Luistro A, Samartino L: Treatment of contact lens-induced giant papillary conjunctivitis, *Cont Lens Assoc Ophthalmol J* 10:346-351, 1984.
21. Orsborn G, Robboy M: Hydrogel lenses and dry-eye symptoms, *Trans Br Cont Lens Assoc Ann Clin Conf* 6:37-38, 1989.
22. Efron N, Golding TR, Brennan NA: The effect of soft lens lubricants on symptoms and lens dehydration, *Cont Lens Assoc Ophthalmol J* 17:114-119, 1991.
23. Golding TR, Efron N, Brennan NA: Soft lens lubricants and prelens tear film stability, *Optom Vis Sci* 67:461-465, 1990.
24. Carney LG, Fullard RJ: Ocular irritation and environmental pH, *Aust J Optom* 62:335, 1979.
25. Fletcher EL, Brennan NA: The effect of solution tonicity on the eye, *Clin Exp Optom* 76:17-21, 1993.
26. Paugh JP, Brennan NA, Efron N: Ocular response to hydrogen peroxide, *Am J Optom Physiol Opt* 65:91-98, 1988.
27. Gyulai P, Dziabo A, Kelly W, Kiral R, Powell CH: Relative neutralization ability of six hydrogen peroxide disinfection solutions, *Cont Lens Spectrum* 2:61-68, 1987.
28. Efron N, Brennan NA, Sek B: Wearing patterns with HEMA contact lenses, *Int Cont Lens Clin* 15:344-350, 1988.

Index

Soft contact lenses–cont'd
  power changes in
    causing vision loss, 126-127
    from flexure, 126
  protocols with, HIV and, 18
  vs. spectacles, 131
  spherical low water content,
      therapeutic tinting and, 109
  surface deposits on, reduced visual
      acuity with, 128-129, 129
  therapeutically tinted
    fitting procedures for, 109-111
    vs. tinted RGP contact lenses, 111-112
  thicker, vision affected by, 128
  tight
    conjunctival trauma from, 75
    corneal infiltrates with, 64
    corneal vascularization and, 73
  toric, with epitheliopathy, 26, 37
  visual problems with, 123-126
    characterization of, 136
    eye factors causing, 131-135
    lens factors causing, 128-131
  in warm climates, ulcerative keratitis
      with, 68
Soft gel lenses; see also Hydrogel contact
      lenses
  therapeutically tinted
    for cataractogenesis, 118
    for Fuch's corneal dystrophy, 118
Soft lens extended-wear, 51-82; see also
      Hydrogel extended-wear lenses
  Acanthamoeba keratitis with, 12
  discontinuation of
    CLPC causing, 70
    GPC causing, 70
  epithelial microcysts with, 90
  lens adherence with, 99
  maximum wear time for, 52
Solution hypersensitivity; see also
      Solution sensitivity
  as contact lens complication, 2
Solution preservatives
  adverse reactions to, with dry eye
      conditions, 24
  affecting CLPC, 70
  causing CLSLK, 78
  causing vision loss, 133
  immunological reaction to
    causing corneal infiltrates, 150
    CLSLK and, 151

Solution preservatives–cont'd
  in lens care systems, CLARE and, 66
  residual, ocular discomfort from, 153
  solution sensitivity and, 74
Solution sensitivity, 74-75
  causing corneal vascularization, 73
  corneal infiltrates with, 64
Solutions; see Lens care solutions
Spatial disruptions, with
      color–vision-altering devices, 108
Spectacle blur
  after polymethyl methacrylate lenses
      removal, 112
  with corneal distortion, from lens
      adherence, 97
  with lens adherence, 100
Spectacles
  with contact lenses, for presbyopia
      correction, 127
  vs. soft contact lenses, 131
  tinted, vs. tinted contact lens
      correction, 113
Specular reflection
  for bleb response observation, 59
  for corneal exhaustion syndrome
      observation, 60
  for endothelium polymegethism
      observation, 59
Specular reflex, conjunctival
  normal appearance of, 32
  tear deficiencies affecting, 32
SPK; see Superficial punctate keratitis (SPK)
Staining
  with conjunctival trauma, 75, 77
  corneal; see Corneal staining
  fluorescein; see Fluorescein staining
  4-8 o'clock; see 4-8 o'clock staining
  instillation of
    observations following, 33
    in tear deficiency biomicroscopic
        sequence, 32, 33
  lid closure; see 3-9 o'clock staining
  limbal; see Limbal staining
  pinpoint, with epithelial cell loss, 95
  punctate
    with Acanthamoeba keratitis, 13
    with RGP extended wear, 95
  3-9 o'clock; see 3-9 o'clock staining
Staphylococcal blepharitis, 6-9
  chronic, 7
    contact lens prescriptions with, 8